Percutaneous Lumbar Discectomy

Edited by
H. Michael Mayer and Mario Brock

With 134 Figures

Springer-Verlag Berlin Heidelberg New York
London Paris Tokyo Hong Kong

Dr. H. MICHAEL MAYER

Professor Dr. Dr. h.c. MARIO BROCK

Universitätsklinikum Steglitz
Neurochirurgische Klinik
Hindenburgdamm 30
1000 Berlin 45, FRG

ISBN 3-540-51032-X Springer-Verlag Berlin Heidelberg New York
ISBN 0-387-51032-X Springer-Verlag New York Berlin Heidelberg

Library of Congress Cataloging-in-Publication Data. Percutaneous lumbar discectomy / edited by H. Michael Mayer and Mario Brock. p. cm. Includes index. ISBN 0-387-51032-X (U.S.: alk. paper) 1. Discectomy. 2. Vertebrae, Lumbar – Surgery. I. Mayer, H. Michael (Heinz-Michael), II. Brock, M. (Mario). [DNLM: 1. Intervertebral Disk–surgery. 2. Lumbar Vertebrae–surgery. WE 750 P429] RD771.I6P47 1989 617.5′6–dc20 DNLM/DLC for Library of Congress.

Typesetting, printing and bookbinding: Konrad Triltsch, Graphischer Betrieb, Würzburg
2122/3130-543210 – Printed on acid-free paper

List of Contributors

Adresses are given at the beginning of the respective contribution

Preface

It has always been, and still is, one of the major aims of surgery to achieve the best therapeutic effect with the least iatrogenic trauma. This goal was attained in an unprecedented way by the application of microsurgical techniques to neurosurgery and of arthroscopic procedures to orthopedic surgery. The treatment of lumbar disc disease, however, has not benefited from such advances for many years. Modern imaging methods have set the stage for a selective therapeutic approach to herniated lumbar discs. Among the new and alternative surgical procedures, percutaneous lumbar discectomy (PLD) is the youngest child. Since its first description by Hijikata in 1975, several techniques for the percutaneous removal of herniated lumbar disc material have been developed: PLD with forceps and shaver systems, PLD with endoscopic control (discoscopy), automated PLD (APLD) using disposable nucleotome probes, percutaneous endoscopic laser discectomy (PELD) and even PLD with bone grafting. Despite these revolutionary developments, however, there are still uncertainties concerning patient selection, indications, surgical technique, results, post-operative management and potential hazards. For this reason, experts in the field of percutaneous discectomy gathered at an international symposium in Berlin on August 12 and 13, 1988, to share their experience and to present the "state of the art" of this procedure. This volume contains the major contributions to the symposium. We hope it may serve as a reference work for future clinical and experimental studies.

Berlin

H. Michael Mayer
Mario Brock

Contents

History

Anatomy

Pathophysiology

Diagnosis

Percutaneous Lumbar Discectomy (PLD) – Technique and Results

Automated Percutaneous Lumbar Discectomy (APLD)

Experimental Approaches and Perspectives

History

History of Surgical Treatment of Herniated Lumbar Discs

P. KAMBIN [1]

A review of the history of the surgical treatment of herniated lumbar discs would not be complete without paying tribute to the numerous scientists, researchers and clinicians who have contributed to the understanding of the pathophysiology and anatomical structures of the intervertebral disc, the clinical manifestation of root compression due to abnormally protruded disc and its myelographic, CT and MRI diagnosis.

Mixter and Barr [14] deserve credit for their detailed description of a herniated lumbar disc as an etiological factor for root compression and sciatica. Their well-documented publication in 1934 contributed to the popularization and acceptance of laminectomy for the decompression of the spinal canal and extraction of the disc fragments.

Prior to that, a number of reports indicating the discovery of disc herniation and its surgical extraction had appeared in the medical literature. Virchow [27], in 1858, described his autopsy findings on an intervertebral disc in a patient who expired following severe trauma. Calling it a fractured disc, he elaborated on its microscopic and gross appearance. Goldthwait [8], in 1911, described the history and findings of a 39-year-old male whose low back pain was attributed to sacroiliac displacement. This patient developed paraparesis in the course of manipulation of the sacroiliac joint and plaster immobilization. Six weeks later, due to lack of improvement, he was submitted to extensive laminectomy from L1 to S2. During the surgery, no pathology was found except the narrowing of the canal at the lumbosacral junction. The neurological status of the patient subsequently improved but he continued to exhibit pain. Goldthwait attributed the development of the neurological changes in the lower extremities to instability produced by slippage of the articular processes, abnormalities of the transverse process of the fifth lumbar vertebra and the detachment of the annulus from the vertebral plates and its protrusion into the spinal canal.

In the early 20th century, laminectomy was being performed for the decompression of the spinal canal and in some cases, for the relief of sciatic pain. Elsberg (1913) and Dandy (1929) reported extraction from the canal a fibrocartilaginous tissue causing compression of the neural structures [4, 5]. In 1928, Alajouanine [1], a neurologist in Paris, reported the extraction of a herniated disc in a 20-year-old female patient who demonstrated a motor deficit and had positive Lipiodol myelography.

[1] The Graduate Hospital, Disc Treatment and Research Center, University of Pennsylvania, School of Medicine, Philadelphia, PA 19104, USA

Percutaneous Lumbar Discectomy
Ed. by H. M. Mayer and M. Brock

The search for an alternative method of treatment for herniated lumbar discs began in the 1950s. Hult [10], in 1951, reported on his experience of anterolateral decompression of the herniated lumbar discs through a retroperitoneal approach. The introduction of chemonucleolysis by Lyman Smith [24] provided us with the concept that a herniated disc can be treated by an indirect approach without the need for visualization and extraction of the herniated site. Prior to this publication, Thomas [25] reported the utilization of papain in rabbits and demonstrated the softening and drop of the rabbits' ears.

Love [12], in 1939, and Williams [28], in 1979, described their experience in microlumbar discectomy, which allows access to the spinal canal through a small incision for the removal of disc fragments.

The percutaneous approach to the lumbar intervertebral discs represents a new concept in the treatment of protruded symptom-producing discs. In contrast to laminectomy or microlumbar discectomy, the spinal canal and its content is not violated in the course of this procedure.

Great tribute should be paid to Valls [26], Ottolenghi [19] and Craig [3] for their work and publications on the posterolateral approach to the spine. Although this procedure was principally described for biopsy purposes, the approach was later utilized for discography, chemonucleotherapy and subsequently for percutaneous lumbar discectomy. Ottolenghi's schematic drawing demonstrating the proper positioning of the needle via the posterolateral approach has remained unchallenged.

Our experimental work with percutaneous lumbar discectomy began in 1973 [11]. Our first patient was a 60-year-old male with right sciatica who had a disc protrusion at the L3–4 and L4–5 levels. The L3–4 disc was excised following laminectomy, while the L4–5 disc was decompressed and partially evacuated through a Craig cannula inserted dorsolaterally.

A 43-year-old female with a clinical and myelographic diagnosis of L4–5 disc herniation was submitted to percutaneous lumbar discectomy in April of 1974; however, we were unable to reach the posterior fragments. This patient subsequently required laminectomy for the removal of the sequestrated disc material.

In June of 1974, a 37-year-old male with persistent low back pain and left sciatica was admitted to the hospital. His myelogram showed disc herniations at the L4–5 and L5–S1 levels. Both levels were explored surgically, and a large herniation found at L5–S1 was excised. The L4–5 disc was partially evacuated utilizing a Craig cannula and small punch forceps.

In February of 1974, a similar operation was performed on a 52-year-old male with right sciatic pain and myelographic evidence of disc herniation at both L3–4 and L4–5 levels. A large herniation at L4–5 was found and extracted following bilateral hemilaminectomy. The L3–4 level was decompressed and partially evacuated with a Craig cannula inserted via the percutaneous approach.

Our subsequent experimental work in cadavers proved the safety of forced suction in the intervertebral discs. From the pathological examination of the intervertebral discs in fresh cadavers, we learned the necessity of developing the technology which would allow us to reach posteriorly and evacuate the symptom-producing fragment in certain patients.

In October of 1980, our preliminary experience and plans for the future treatment of patients with herniated lumbar discs by the percutaneous method was submitted to the Human Subject Committee of The Graduate Hospital, University of Pennsylvania, School of Medicine, for approval. The appropriate documentation for patient information and education was developed. Subsequently nine patients were treated under a strict protocol by this method. The detailed clinical and myelographic findings, operative technique and results were subsequently published in the *Journal of Clinical Orthopaedics and Related Research* [11]. To the best of our knowledge, this was the first report in a medical journal with worldwide distribution. Dr. Hijikata [9] should be credited for his independent work on percutaneous nucleotomy in 1975 and his fine report in the *Journal of Toden Hospital* in Japan.

Friedman [7] in 1983, reported his experience with the introduction of a 40-French chest tube and speculum into the intervertebral discs through a 1-in. (2.5-cm) incision over the iliac crest. Due to the far lateral approach and the size of the instruments, several complications have been encountered in the course of this operative procedure. Schreiber [22] and Suezawa (biportal approach and discoscopy of the intervertebral discs) and Monteiro [15] (emphasis of posterolateral hole decompression of the intervertebral disc) deserve credit for their contributions. Onik [18] et al. have introduced an automated instrument for nuclear evacuation.

The scientists, researchers and clinicians who have contributed to the progress of disc surgery are too many to mention in this brief summary. Great tribute should be paid to Roentgen, a German physicist, for the discovery of x-ray. Lipiodol myelography introduced by Sicard and Forestier [23], subsequently led to the discovery of metrizamide and other water-soluble radiopaque material and opened the way to the diagnosis and isolation of symptom-producing discs.

The contributions of Radon [21], Oldendorf [16, 17], Cromak and Hounsfield, who subsequently, in 1979, shared a Nobel prize for medicine for the development of the CT scan, deserve recognition.

The scientists who have contributed to the development of MRI are too numerous to list by name. Block [2] and Purcell [20], who shared a Nobel prize on this subject, should be remembered.

The contributions of Farfan [6] to the understanding of the biomechanics of intervertebral discs and MacNab [13] in degenerative changes of intervertebral discs also deserve credit.

The scientists of our time whose work keeps the flame of progress lit, both in the field of disc surgery and in the pathophysiology of the nerve root and the spinal nerve, are likewise too many to mention, and for this I extend my apologies.

References

1. Alajouanine TH (1978) From the presidential address by Professor Jean Cauchoix before annual meeting of the Internat'l. Soc. for the study of the lumbar spine, San Francisco, Cal., June 1978

2. Block F (1946) Nuclear induction. Physiol Rev 70:460
3. Craig FS (1956) Vertebral body biopsy. J Bone Joint Surg 38A:93
4. Dandy WE (1929) Loose cartilage from intervertebral disk simulating tumor of the spinal cord. Arch Surg 19:660
5. Elsberg CA (1913) Experiences in spinal surgery: Observations upon 60 laminectomies for spinal disease. Surg Gynec Obstet 16:117
6. Farfan HF (1973) Mechanical disorders of the low back. Lea & Febiger, Philadelphia
7. Friedman WA (1983) Percutaneous discectomy: An alternative to chemonucleolysis. J Neurosurg 13:542
8. Goldthwait JE (1911) The lumbosacral articulation: An explanation of many cases of "lumbago", "sciatica" and paraplegia. Boston Med Surg J. 164:365
9. Hijikata SA (1975) A method of percutaneous nuclear extraction. J Toden Hospital 5:39
10. Hult L (1951) Retroperitoneal disc fenestration in low back pain and sciatica. Acta Orthop Scand 20:3423
11. Kambin P, Gellman H (1983) Percutaneous lateral discectomy of the lumbar spine: A preliminary report. Clin Orthop 174:127
12. Love JG (1939) Removal of protruded intervertebral discs without laminectomy. Proc Staff Meeting, Mayo Clinic 14:800
13. MacNab I (1952) Disc degeneration and low back pain. Royal College of Phys. and Surg. of Canada Annual Meeting Proceedings 3 and 4, Oct. 1952
14. Mixter WJ, Barr JS (1934) Rupture of the intervertebral disc with involvement of the spinal canal. N Engl J Med 211:210
15. Monteiro A (1987) Percutaneous lumbar discectomy. International Symposium, Graduate Hospital, University of Pa., March 1987
16. Oldendorf WH (1961) Displaying the internal structural pattern of a complex object. Ir Trans Bio-Med Elect BME 8:68
17. Oldendorf WH (1980) The quest for an image of the brain. Raven, New York
18. Onik G, Helms C, Ginsberg L, Hoaglund T, Morris J (1985) Percutaneous lumbar discectomy using a new aspiration probe. AJNR 6:290
19. Ottolenghi CE (1955) Vertebral body biopsy, aspiration biopsy. Jour B & J Surg 37-A, June 1955
20. Purcell EM et al. (1946) Resonance absorption by nuclear magnetic moments in a solid. Phys Rev 69:37–38
21. Radon: Quoted by Oldendorf WH (1980) The quest for an image of the brain. Raven, New York
22. Schreiber A, Suezawa Y (1986) Transdiscoscopic percutaneous nucleotomy in disc herniation. Orthop Rev 15:75
23. Sicard JA, Forestier J (1921) Methode radiographique d'exploration de la cavité epidurale par le Lipiodal. Rev Neurol 37:1264
24. Smith L (1963) Enzyme dissolution of the intervertebral disc. Nature 4887:198
25. Thomas L (1956) Reversible collapse of rabbit ears after intravenous papain. J Exp Med 104:245
26. Valls J, Ottolenghi CE, Schajowicz F (1948) Aspiration biopsy in diagnosis of lesions of vertebral bodies. JAMA 136:376
27. Virchow R (1857) Untersuchungen über die Entwickelung des Schädelgrundes. Reimer, Berlin
28. Williams RW (1979) Microsurgical lumbar discectomy. Report to American Association of Neurology and Surgery 1975. Neurosurgery 4(2):140

Anatomy

Anatomy of the Posterolateral Spine

J. A. N. SHEPPERD [1]

Introduction

The safety and efficacy of percutaneous back surgery depends on understanding the anatomy. Between the skin which the surgeon sees and the bones which the x-rays show, a great deal is otherwise left to guesswork. The relevant anatomy is not adequately covered in standard texts and we, therefore, undertook a series of 40 cadaver dissections (reported in two separate papers at the British Society for Back Pain Research in 1980 and 1981).

The lateral nerve root was studied at individual segments of the spine as it passed below the pedicles and through the exit foramen. This part of the root is not seen at conventional surgery. Soft tissue, laminae and pedicles were systematically removed so that the roots were displayed fully. Measurements were taken in the subfacet region and also between the disc and intertransverse ligaments as the root passed distally. Finally, the theca was filled with methylene blue and measurements made of the extent of the thecal covering along the nerve root. Based on these studies I intend to cover four topics in this chapter. (A) The general anatomy, (B) The posterolateral anatomy, (C) The anatomy of the disc, and (D) Radiological landmarks.

General Anatomy

A useful concept is an axial slice of the trunk, parallel with the disc and between the upper end plate of a lumbar vertebra and the upper end plate of the vertebra below. The section indicates how centrally the spinal structures lie with approximately two-thirds in the posterior abdominal wall and one-third in the back. Such a slice includes inferior and superior facet joint components of the vertebrae above and below respectively. The skeletal arrangement is well visualised on x-ray and readily revised on a skeleton but is of least importance to the percutaneous surgeon in the sense that it can not be damaged. At risk structures are invisible. These include: 1) the exiting nerve root, 2) the theca, 3) the ilio-lumbar vasculature, particularly venous drainage, and 4) the viscera in the retroperitoneal space.

[1] Hastings Orthopaedic Centre, Royal East Sussex Hospital Hastings, East Sussex TN34 1ER, England

Percutaneous Lumbar Discectomy
Ed. by H. M. Mayer and M. Brock

All these can and have been damaged by the postero-lateral approach and will be considered individually.

1. Exiting nerve root. As the nerve courses down passing the lateral recess and in close proximity with the medial and then inferior wall of the pedicle, it gradually loses its thecal covering. The extent to which the theca is patent in this area was variable in the specimens studied but a degree of tethering on the anterior surface of the root was noticed quite commonly as it turned the corner. This appears to be a normal anatomical feature and not due to scarring from pathological processes. The extent to which the thecal sac is patent in this part of the root sheath once again was variable, but only reached the lower border of the pedicle in 50%. From this position the nerve root moves well laterally and crosses the disc at an angle of between 40–45° in both the AP and lateral views. Only in exceptional circumstance would it be at risk from a disc prolapse or facet impingement at this lower level, despite the fact that comment is often passed regarding x-ray appearance of the exit foramen. It is the medially placed descending root which is at risk of impingement in the lateral recess from either disc or facet joint.
2. The theca. The possibility of damaging the dural sheath undoubtedly exists and is dependent on the extent of the thecal sheath along its root canal. Also the size of the superior facet and its ability, therefore, to protect the main thecal sheath over the descending root. It is more usual that the theca is protected from the postero-lateral approach but anatomical variations occur. The use of curved approach systems would increase the risk of thecal penetration. These aspects warrant careful consideration of pre-operative CT scans.
3. The ilio-lumbar arterial and particularly venous systems are highly vascular and in close proximity to the exiting root and paravertebral structures. Damage to small veins in this area is extremely common but usually of a minor nature. A dull ended initial probe reduces the risk of transfixing a vessel, and close fitting coaxial access tubes minimise risk of laceration. Nevertheless, significant haemorrhage is a possibility and should be considered in the post operative care of these patients.
4. The exit foramen and subfacet region are anterior to the transverse process and in the same coronal plane as the posterior abdominal wall. Technically this is, therefore, in the retroperitoneal space, although in the upper lumbar spine the psoas muscle intervenes and offers some protection. The attachment of psoas and its migration laterally means that at the L 5/S 1 level in particular the instrumentation is in the open retroperitoneal space and close proximity to the viscera. A vertical approach or misinterpretation of x-rays is quite capable of producing penetration of bowel, particularly the sigmoid colon on the left. Damage to great vessels is less likely than at conventional open surgery because of the x-ray control employed.

Postero-Lateral Anatomy

The postero-lateral oblique view will be described in slightly more detail because it provides a concept of the view which would be seen by an advancing percu-

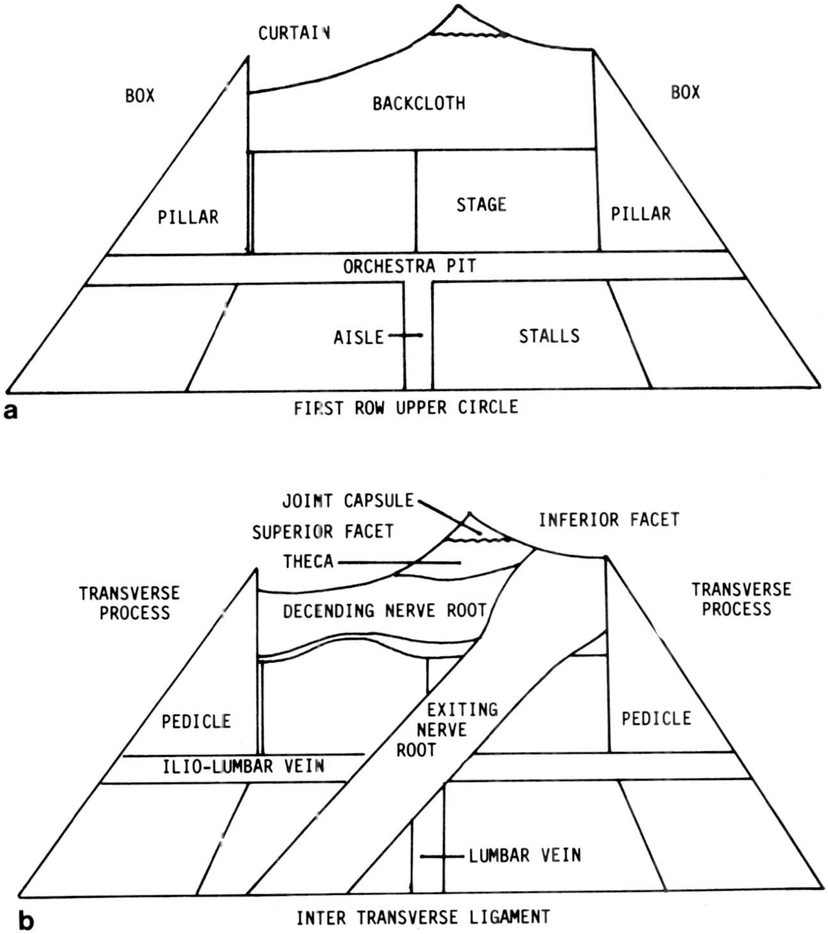

Fig. 1. **a** Stylized view of theatre interior seen from the upper circle. **b** Analogous arrangement of the anatomy of a lateral spinal passage of a right lumbar nerve root, viewed from the 45° posterolateral position used for percutaneous access. Anterior to the transverse process is the retroperitoneal space with vital structures which can be damaged: the approach should aim at "X" posterior to the exiting root and anterior to the descending root, which is usually affected by disc protrusion

taneous instrument. We have defined the lateral spinal passage of a lumbar nerve root as from the caudal border of its named pedicle to the cephalic anterior surface of the transverse process below (or alar of the sacrum for L 5). It lies in the retro-peritoneal space. Viewed from a 45° posterolateral position, the arrangement resembles the inside of a theatre (Fig. 1) as seen from the upper circle, whose front row is the intertransverse ligament and whose boxes to the left and right are the medial ends of the transverse processes. These connect with two pillars (the pedicles) at either side of the stage. For a right nerve root passage, the stage is the vertebral body (right half) and intervertebral disc (left half). The

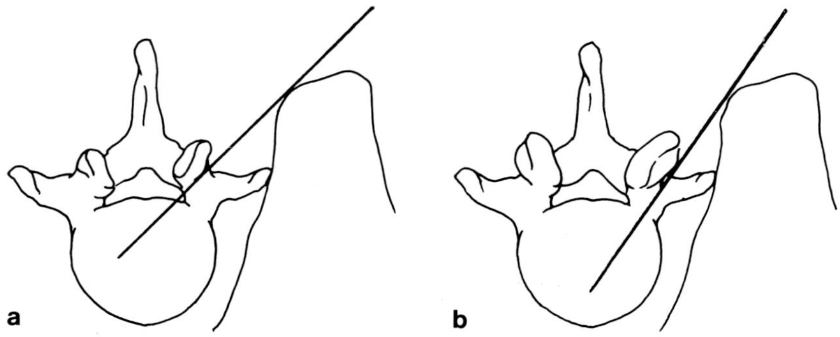

Fig. 2a, b. The line of approach for a probe will depend on height of iliac wing in combination with size of superior facet

backcloth is the theca and the vaulted roof is formed by the superior and inferior facets, with the joint capsule suspended where they meet. The stalls are divided by an aisle (lumbar vein) draining into an orchestra pit (ilio-lumbar vein) in front of the stage. A considerable portion of the back stalls is occupied by the common iliac vein with the artery beneath and other retroperitoneal structures deep in the basement. The star of the show is the emerging root entering from the right wing with its dorsal root ganglion obliterating the back cloth next to the pedicle. Cloaked in a venous plexus, it crosses diagonally to the front of the stage and then over the orchestra pit to disappear below the left box. The root below is seen exiting stage left into the wings and may be negotiating a disc herniation (since it is the root most commonly affected by a prolapsed disc). This leaves the left hand side of the stage (mainly intervertebral disc) virtually clear, even more so if the spine and legs are flexed, when the emerging root has reduced tension and is drawn slightly forward by the transverse process (or ala of the sacrum). A spotlight from the back of the stage is projected onto this bare area in anticipation of the other characters in the percutaneous show: the access tubes and instruments. The exit foramen varies. Variables include the size of facet joint, the distance between the lower end plate and pedicle and the size and height of disc and size of root (Figs. 2, 3). If the disc is narrow the root is brought further distally leaving less space. This may be as a result of variations in normal anatomy or due to degenerative change. Awareness of these aspects should be taken into account when considering both CT scans and plain x-rays.

Disc Anatomy

The anatomy of a disc nucleus is more structured than commonly indicated. It is affected by three factors – 1) the physical properties of proteoglycans which causes the anatomy to change according to activity and circadian rhythm; 2) the dynamic changes which occur in flexion, extension and loading; 3) changes with age. The annular layers in the front of the disc are robust and organised whereas

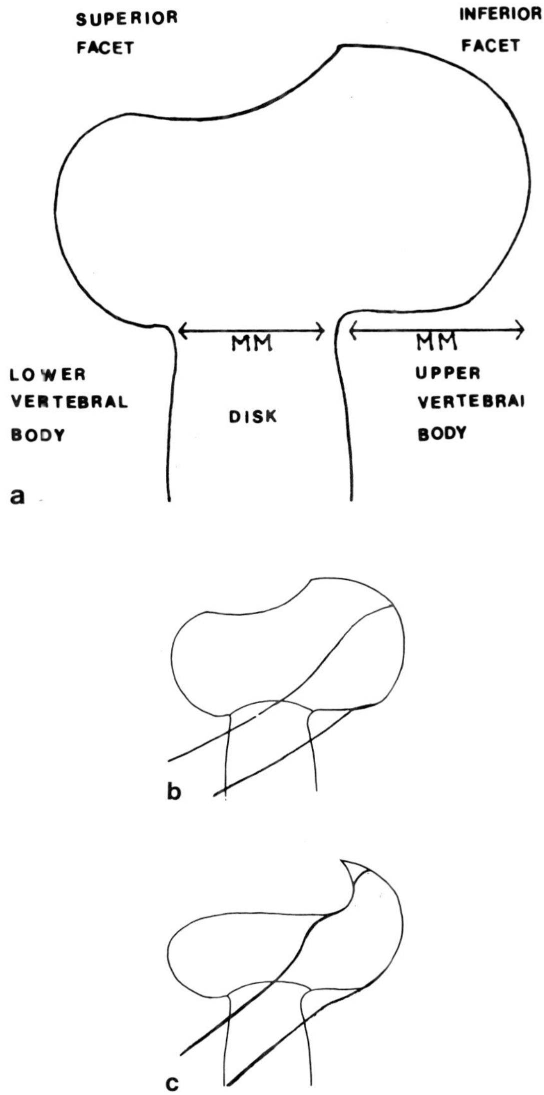

Fig. 3a–c. Normal variations. The ratio of disc height to the bone from lower end plate of the vertebra to the lower edge of the same vertebra's pedicle was variable (between 10/10 and 5/15). The free space for nerve root was also measured and ranged from 5 mms to no free space at all. The reasons include variations in nerve root diameter and variations in size of exit foramen

the annular layers in the posterior disc are more attenuated. Although only the peripheral annulus has nerve fibres, the posterior longitudinal ligament with its lateral expansion is highly innervated and sensitive. The nucleus of the disc is not a simple homogeneous structure. In the centre it is more fluid containing relatively little collagen and further peripherally the collagen content increases. There is no point where it suddenly becomes annulus but particularly posteriorly a gradual gradation is found. The collagen in the nucleus attaches to end plate cartilage so that in early life the whole structure of the nucleus is tethered. When this tethering fails it can cause nuclear material to herniate. Disc herniations may

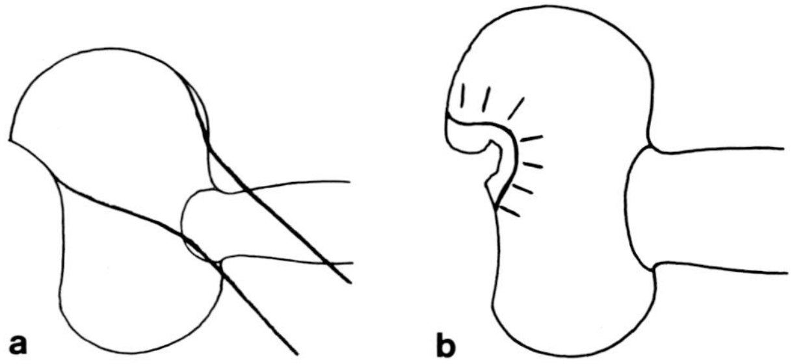

Fig. 4a, b. Ageing changes. **a** Narrow of disc space produces bulging of the annulus combined with cephalad advancement of the superior facet and thereby reduction in the root space foramen ratio. **b** Facet joint arthritis may produce an effusion and inflammatory swelling of the capsule or peripheral osteophytes to reduce the exit foramen ratio

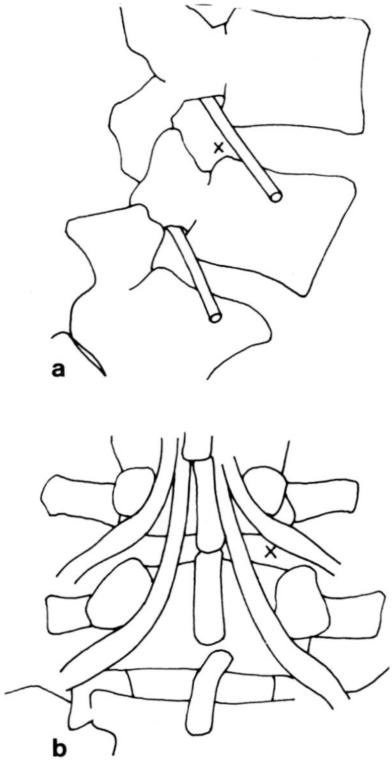

Fig. 5. a Lateral view and **b** AP view of roentgenogram outline showing position of exiting nerve root. The image intensifier tube must be tilted to produce perpendicular projections in both planes. The target for disc entry should be the lower half of the disc in line with the pedicle (AP view) and posterior vertebral body (lateral view) at "X" for L4–5

comprise a detachment of the hard peripheral annulus. Alternatively a peripheral part of the nucleus may get lodged beneath the posterior longitudinal ligament. The proteoglycan-laden nucleus expands and contracts according to the external pressure placed upon it. When a disc has degenerated the proteoglycans are less abundant, the disc loses height. The physical size of nuclear material is dependent on the hydrostatic pressure, and therefore expands greatly when herniated from within the disc.

With ageing, disc compliance and structure alter. We have taken sagittal sections of low lumbar spines in an ageing population and studied the performance of the disc in flexion and extension. Two ageing variations include: 1) increased anterior, posterior movement of nucleus material due to horizontal fissuring, and 2) vertical fissuring which alters the dynamics of the disc and stresses on the facet joint. All these anatomical features of the disc are most important in understanding and properly managing sufferers from disc related disorders.

Radiological Landmarks

It is of paramount importance that AP and lateral projections are obtained parallel with the disc.

Based on the contents of this chapter, and in particular consideration of the anatomical variation which may be encountered, Figures 4 and 5 indicate the ideal radiological landmarks. The instrument should pass caudal to the exiting nerve root. Entry is in line with the pedicle and in the middle to lower half of the disc.

The Posterolateral Approach

J. A. McCulloch [1]

Introduction

Obviously, the passage of large-bore cannulas or the installation of potentially damaging chemicals (e.g. chymopapain) into the lumbar intervertebral disc precludes the use of the midline transdural disc approach. Lindblom [4] first proposed midline discography, and others subsequently popularized the posterolateral or lateral approach to disc puncture [2, 3, 5, 6, 8].

Definitions

Posterior (Midline) Lumbar Discography: Until recently, this was the routine and popular method of puncturing a lumbar disc. Through the midline interspinous/interlaminar route, a needle is inserted across the thecal sac (2 dural punctures; one posterior, the second anterior), between the roots of the cauda equina into the disc space [4].

The Posterolateral Approach: The correct definition of this approach is lateral to the spinous process, but close enough to the midline to enter the interlaminar interval and the disc space (Fig. 1). This approach usually crosses through the axilla of the nerve root and is no longer a viable approach.

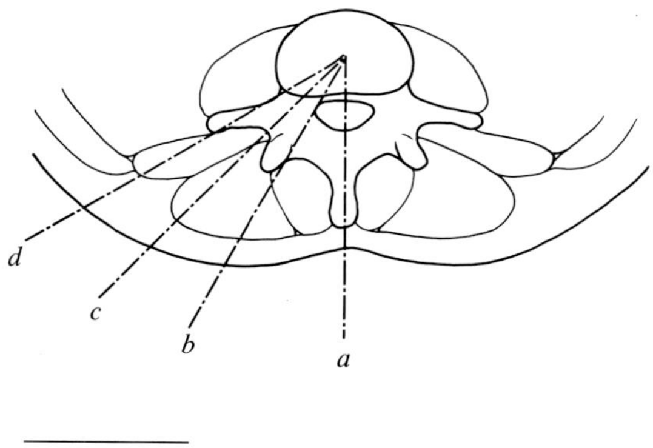

Fig. 1. *Dotted lines* represent the various approaches into disc space: *a* midline, *b* posterolateral that goes through edge of spinal canal, *c* lateral, and *d* far lateral. The last approach, providing it does not transect bowel, is the preferred approach to the disc for percutaneous discectomy. It is about 10 cm from the midline and more than 45 degrees from the sagittal line

[1] Northeastern Ohio Universities College of Medicine, Crystal Clinic, 3975 Embassy Parkway, Suite 102, Akron, OH 44313, USA

Percutaneous Lumbar Discectomy
Ed. by H. M. Mayer and M. Brock

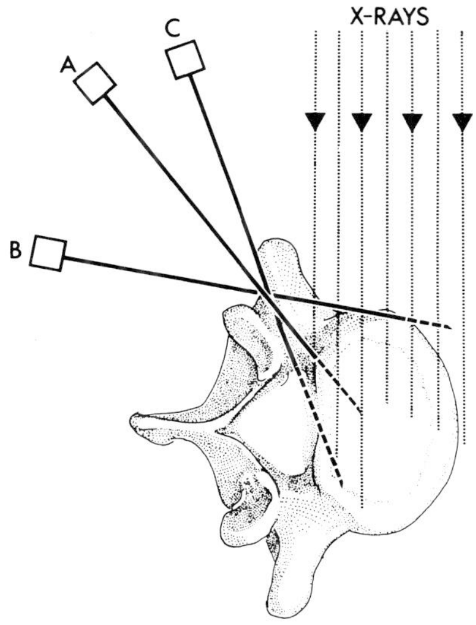

Fig. 2. The lateral approach (*A*). *C* represents an approach too vertical, entering the neural foramen. *B* is an approach too close to the midline and off the edge of the disc space

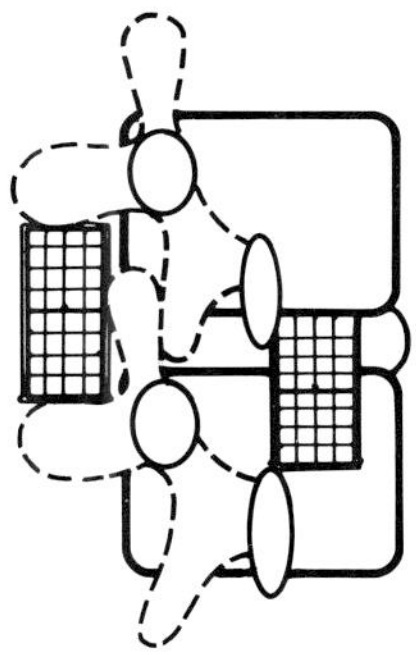

Fig. 3. Windows of opportunity into the spinal canal and disc space. The standard surgical interlaminar window and the lateral intertransverse window

The Lateral Approach: Although this chapter is entitled "The Posterolateral Approach", the author would prefer to think of the approach for percutaneous lumbar discectomy (PLD) as the lateral approach (Fig. 2). The entry to the discal cavity is entirely lateral to the thecal sac and through the intertransverse window (Fig. 3). This approach has turned out to be easier on both the patient and the surgeon and it is becoming the approach of choice for all methods of percutaneous approaches to the disc space, be it for diagnostic or therapeutic purposes. The advantages of this approach are:

1. The only pain-sensitive structures encountered are the skin, periosteum, and, if inadvertently struck, the nerve root. The annulus is relatively insensitive to pain [9].
2. It avoids penetration of the dural sac and inpaling of the cauda equina nerves.

Anatomy of a Lumbar Segment

There are basically two windows of entry into the spinal canal and disc space (Fig. 3):

a) The interlaminar window
b) The intertransverse window

Before describing the approach to each, a brief description of an anatomical segment will be presented. To build an understanding of the anatomy of a lower lumbar segment, take the following steps:

Step 1: Draw an imaginary line at the inferior border of the pedicles (Fig. 4). This divides a vertebral body into an upper half and a lower half.

Step 2: There are three named posterior elements above that line (Fig. 5):
1) pedicle
2) transverse process
3) superior facet

Step 3: There are three named posterior elements below that line (Fig. 6):
1) lamina
2) spinous process
3) inferior facet

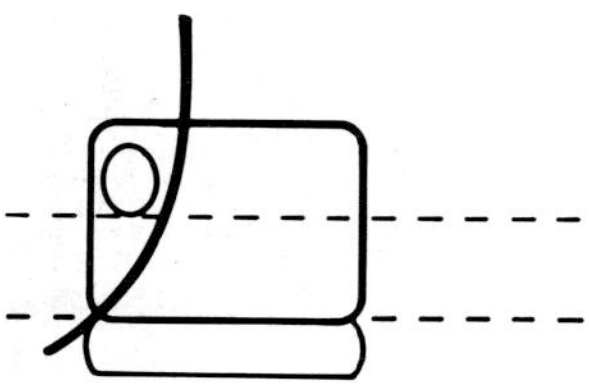

Fig. 4

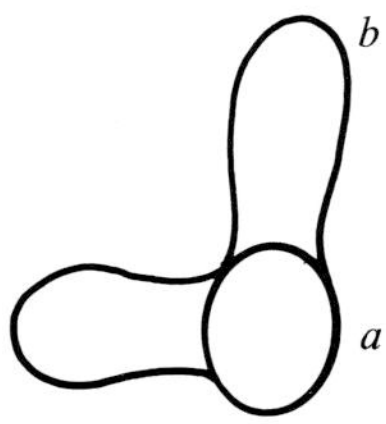

Fig. 5

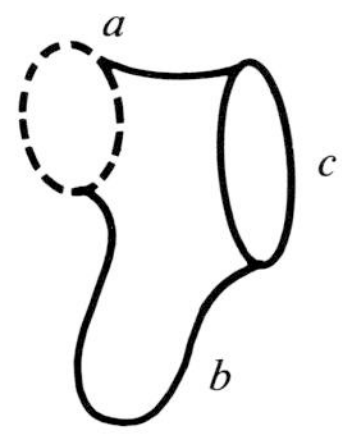

Fig. 6

Fig. 4. A lumbar anatomic segment with its nerve root and an imaginary dotted line at the inferior border of the pedicle

Fig. 5. The three named posterior elements above the line: *a* pedicle, *b* superior facet, *c* transverse process

Fig. 6. The three named posterior elements below the line: a) lamina, b) inferior facet, c) spinous process

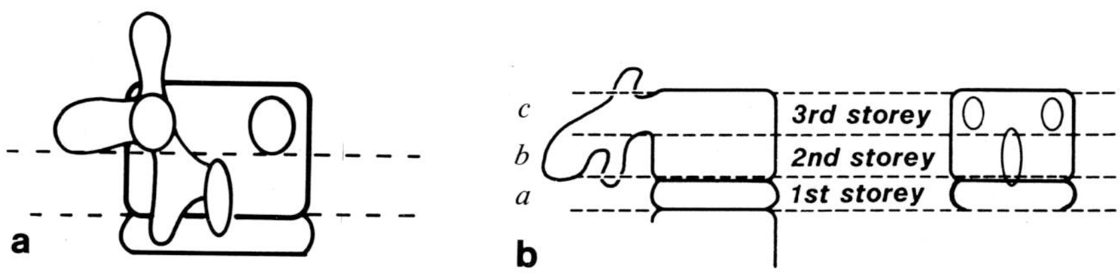

Fig. 7. a The assembled lumbar vertebral anatomic segment. **b** The three-storey concept of skeletal anatomy: *a* the first storey-disc level, *b* the second storey-foraminal level, *c* the third storey-pedicle level

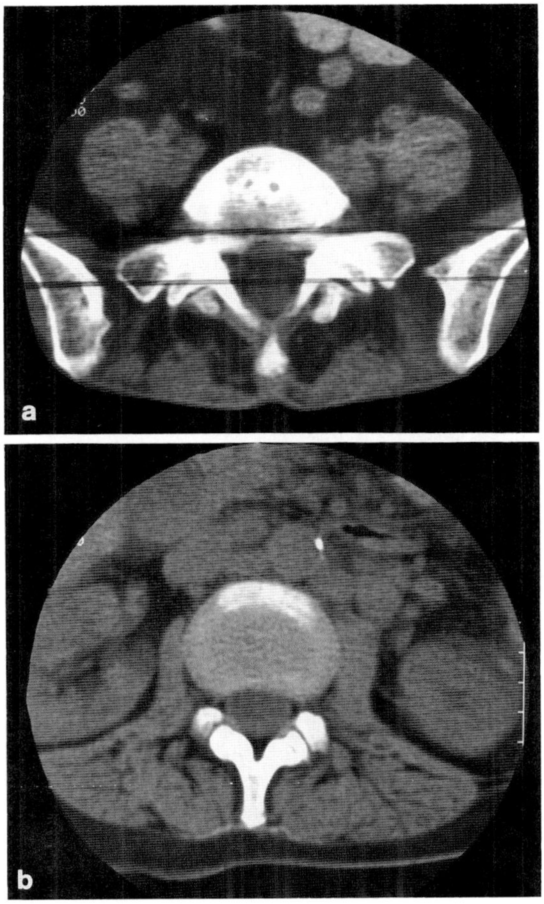

Fig. 8. **a** CT scan showing where you, as reader, should scan to determine which storey slice depicts. This is the 3rd storey of S 1. **b** This is the 1st storey of L 4

Step 4: Joining the three superior elements to the three inferior elements is the pars interarticularis, which lies on the imaginary line joining the inferior borders of the pedicles.

Step 5: Add a disc below (Fig. 7) and you now have a lumbar anatomical segment. Add a vertebra below and the windows of entry to the spinal canal, neurological structures, and disc space are created (Fig. 3).

Step 6: Figure 8 shows how to read a CT scan (or MRI) to know which storey you are in for each slice.

Step 7: Add two nerve roots (Fig. 9):

a) an exiting nerve root

b) a traversing nerve root.

The various figures above demonstrate the three stories that make up each lumbar anatomical segment.

1) the first storey – the disc level

2) the second storey – the foraminal level

3) the third storey – the pedicle level

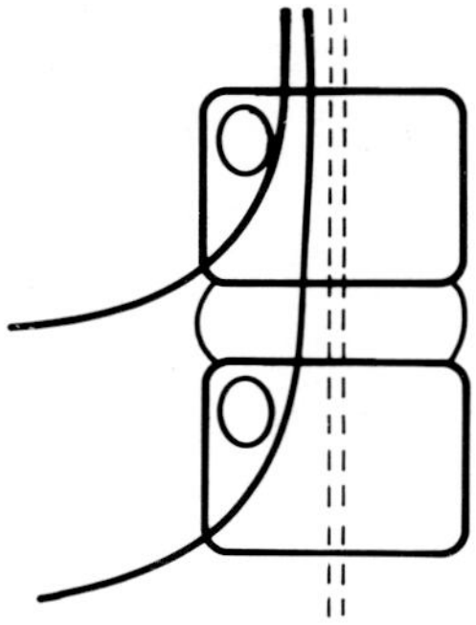

Fig. 9. For the upper anatomic segment the nerve root passing under the pedicle to exit the foramen is known as the exiting nerve root. The root passing by the disc space to exit under the pedicle of the segment below is known as the traversing nerve root

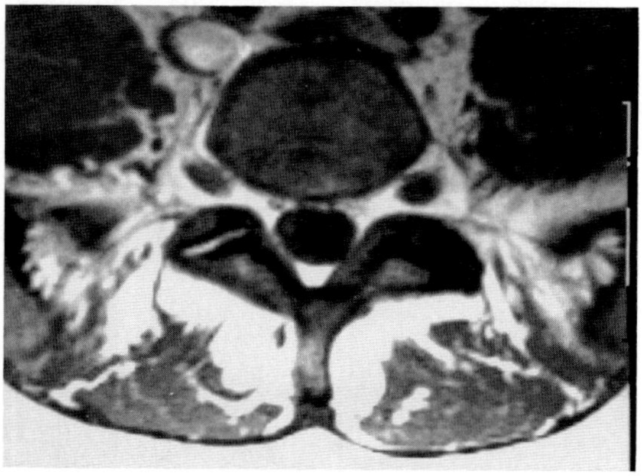

Fig. 10. MRI showing exiting nerve root in foramen of L4, well on its way anteriorly

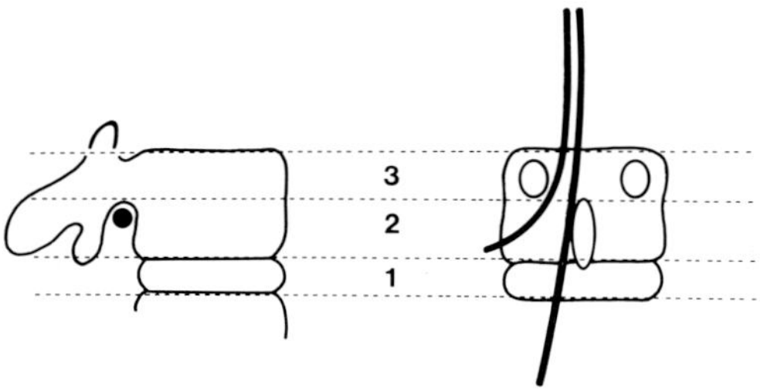

Fig. 11. Three stories with the exiting and traversing nerve roots in place. The window between the two roots is through the intertransverse ligament

Step 8: Note in Fig. 10 that the exiting nerve root, on leaving the foramen, takes an anterior direction. This opens the intertransverse window of opportunity to percutaneous entry to the intradiscal space (Fig. 11).

Anatomy of the Approach

Surgeons are trained in direct hand-eye coordination, allowing them to work in a natural three-dimensional construct. Interpose something between the hand

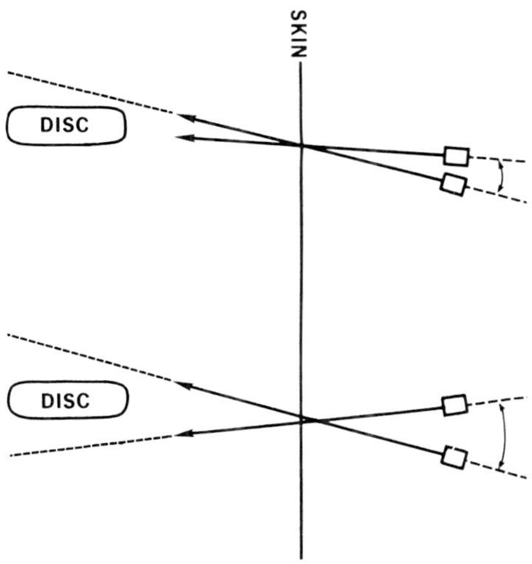

Fig. 12. A slight amount of correction at one end of the needle changes the needle tip direction considerably. It is easy to overcorrect as shown on right-hand drawing

and eye (e.g. a microscope) and, even though three-dimensional viewing is still present, the surgical exercise becomes more difficult. Percutaneous surgery goes one step further – it removes the third dimension and substitutes a two-dimensional x-ray image to guide the surgeon. To adapt to this setting, the surgeon must be constantly adding the third dimension, necessitating the use of simple geometric thinking (Fig. 2).

When trying to place the probe into the disc space, think only of the probe tip in the geometric construct. This prevents overcorrection when redirecting the probe (Fig. 12).

Position of the Patient

During the rise in popularity of chymopapain, most users placed the patient in the lateral position. Percutaneous lumbar discectomy can be done in the lateral position, but to prepare for the advances to be described in this volume, the prone position is recommended as the position of choice because it allows entry from either side or simultaneous entry from each side [7].

Skin Puncture Distance from the Midline

The proper distance from the midline to select for needle puncture is 10 cm in the average 70 kg male. Adjustments less or more from this distance can be made to allow for patient size. Entering closer to the midline will result in the facet joints displacing the probe away from the disc space and entering further from the midline may result in penetration of the viscera (Fig. 13).

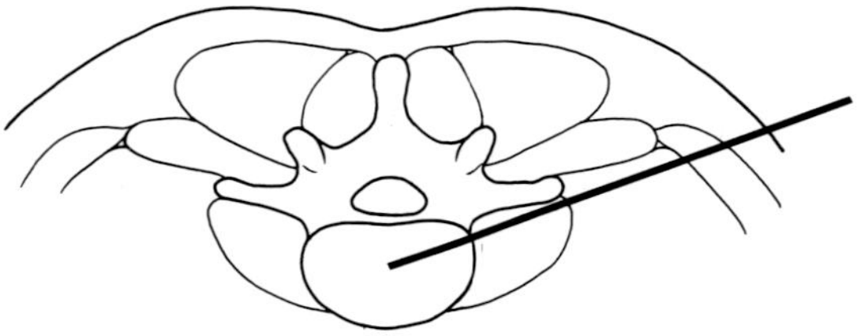

Fig. 13. Too far lateral penetrates the abdominal cavity

Angle of Advancement of the Probe

Selecting a site 10 cm from the midline requires that the probe be advanced at a 50 to 60 degree angle from the horizontal. This allows one to place the probe in the center of the "rectangular disc" (Fig. 14), while avoiding the facet joint behind the probe, the viscera in front of the probe, and the nerve root as it hugs the side of the vertebral body in its anteroinferior course through the psoas.

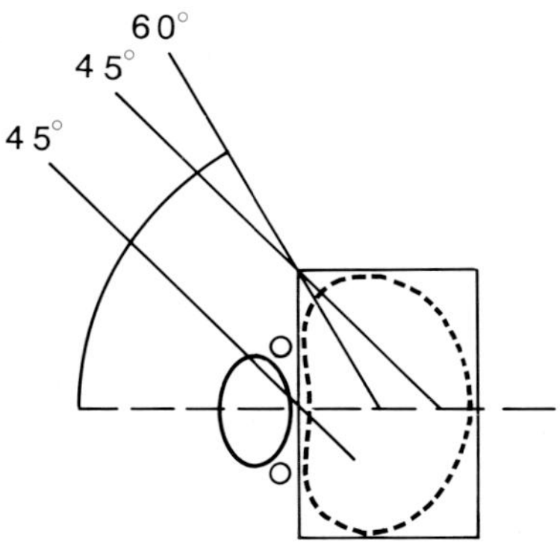

Fig. 14. The correct approach (60°) into the disc cavity that is "rectangular" in shape (especially the L 5 disc)

Bony Obstruction

Remembering the three-stories concept of anatomy for each segment, it is easy to look at Figs. 15 and 16 and see that bony obstruction is occurring in the third storey and must be the superior facet or transverse process. Figure 17 shows other bony obstruction to entry into the disc space.

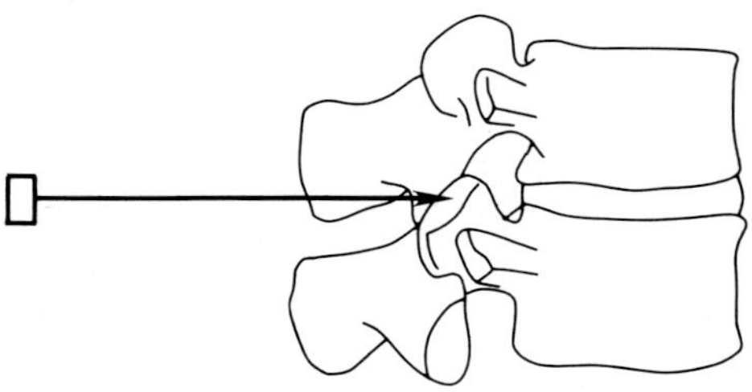

Fig. 15. The probe meeting bony obstruction in the first storey – the superior facet

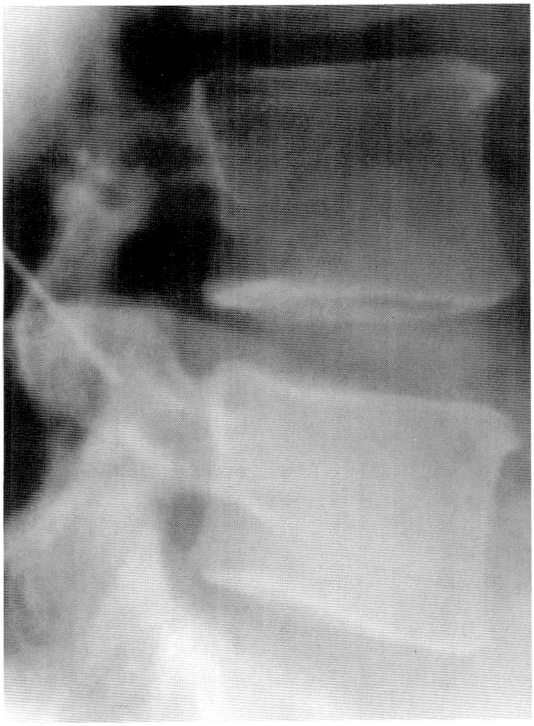

Fig. 16. Image view of obstruction from transverse process

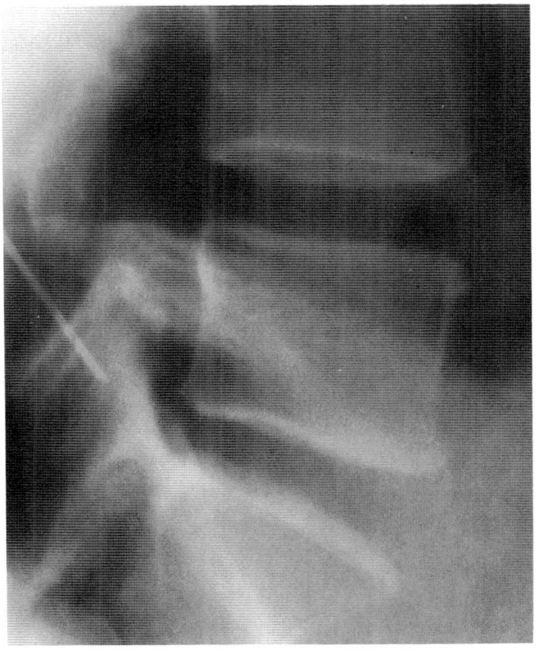

Fig. 17. Bony obstruction opposite the disc space – the facet joint

Entry to Various Levels

It is usually a straight line from the skin entry site to the L4–5 disc and more cephalad discs. Entry to L5–S1 is more difficult because the disc space lies below the intercrestal line, requiring angling of the probe in a caudal direction (30 to 40 degrees).

Positioning of the Probe Tip

Figure 18 shows the three parameters of proper probe tip position.

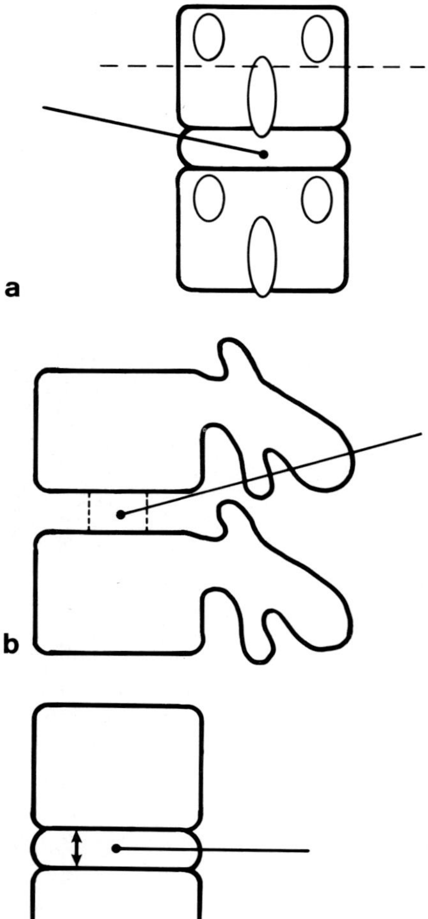

Fig. 18a–c. Proper probe tip positioning. **a** Center of the disc on AP. **b** Center of the disc on lateral (by increasing the angle of approach as in Fig. 14, it is possible to place the probe tip to the posterior aspect of the disc space). **c** Center of the disc cephalad/caudad

Side of Entry

Which side of the patient to enter relative to the pathology and technique has not been discussed in this chapter. Readers are referred to other chapters in this volume for this discussion.

Pitfalls in the Lateral Approach

Wrong Level

The three commonest errors in all of spine surgery are:

1) entry into the wrong level
2) entry into the wrong level
3) entry into the wrong level

The problem of wrong level surgery is far more common than most surgeons are prepared to admit.

Figures 19 and 20 show the two basic errors:

a) selection of the incorrect level
b) misdirection by a radiologist who numbers inappropriately in the face of congenital lumbosacral anomalies

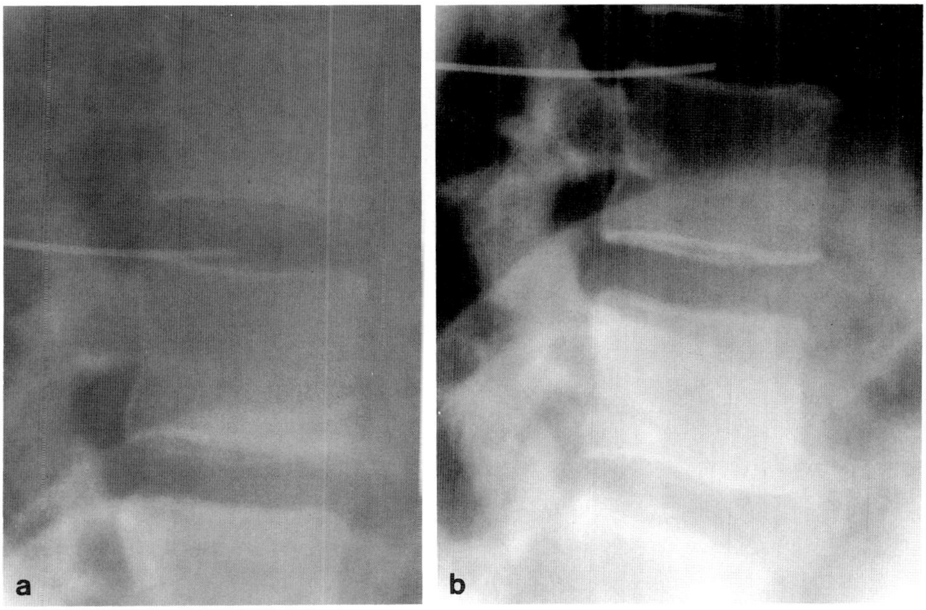

Fig. 19. **a** Is this the L4–5 disc? **b** No, it was the L3–4 disc, discovered by moving the image intensifier caudad to see the L5–S1 junction

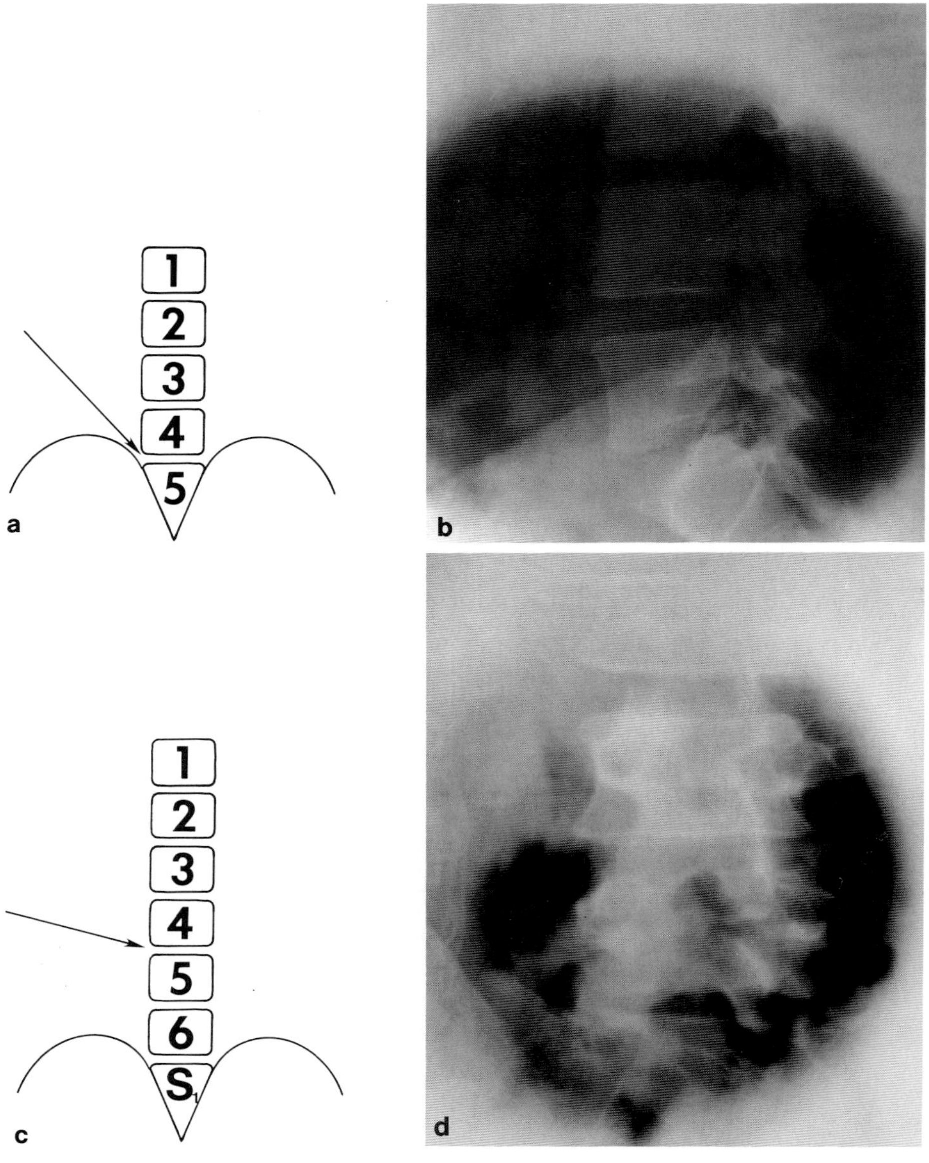

Fig. 20. a Four lumbar vertebrae numbered by the radiologist. **b** The lateral image intensifier view – which space is L4–5? **c** Six lumbar vertebrae numbered by the radiologist. **d** The AP image intensifier view – which space is L4–5?

Scoliosis

On occasion, it is necessary to enter a disc that is part of a scoliotic curve. Figure 21 shows the approach.

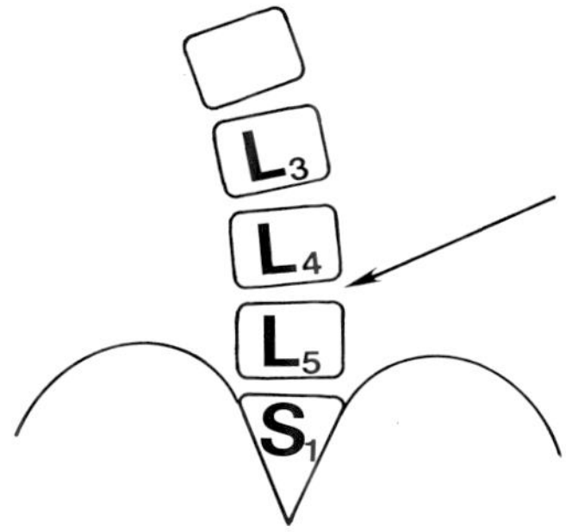

Fig. 21. Always enter from the convex side of a scoliosis

Large Transverse Process of L 5

Usually, a large transverse process of L 5, or a deep set L 5 – S 1, disc space protects the L 5 – S 1 disc space from pathology. There are occasions, however, when it is necessary to enter an L 5 – S 1 disc space with a unilateral large transverse process. Figure 22 shows the method.

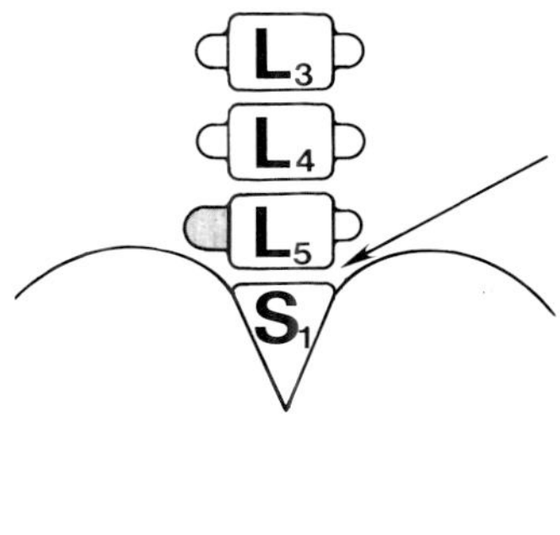

Fig. 22. Enter on the side of the smallest transverse process

Placing the Probe Outside the Pelvis

The experienced user of the lateral approach knows that it is essential to select an entry level at least 1 – 2 cm above the iliac crest to angle down into the L 5 – S 1 disc space. Selecting an entry site too close to the iliac crest will result in the error shown in Fig. 23.

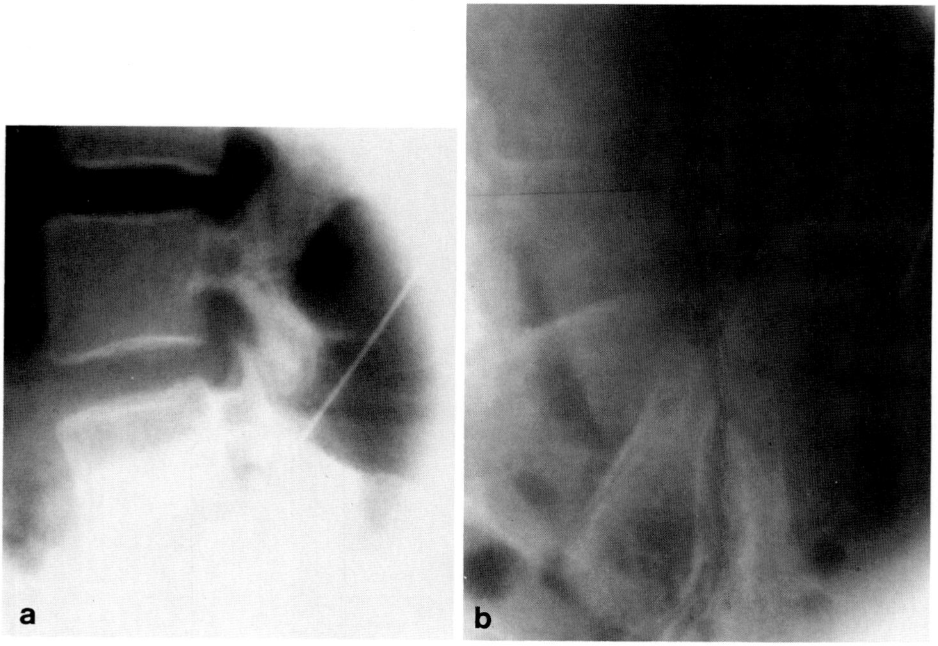

Fig. 23. **a** On lateral, the neddle tip looks good. **b** In the same patient (on AP), the needle is outside of the pelvis – an error made because needle tip selection was too close to the iliac crest

Complications of the Lateral Approach

Penetration of the Nerve Root

With an awake patient, it is difficult to damage the nerve root, providing the approach with the probe is done slowly. If the probe comes in contact with the nerve root, the patient will complain of radicular pain and the probe can be withdrawn and redirected (Fig. 11).

Visceral Injury

Getting too far lateral with the puncture site may result in bowel puncture. Kambin recommends getting a pre-operative CT scan to judge this dimension [2]. Damage to the ureter is usually caused by passing through the other side of the disc space to damage the ureter on the side opposite to entry of the probe.

Great Vessel Injury

At the front of the disc spaces, awaiting the unwary, are the great vessels [1]. Penetration of the L4–5 disc in the midline may injure the aorta and to the right of midline may damage the inferior vena cava. At L5–S1, the iliac arteries and veins are lateral and can be damaged from the opposite side because of penetration of the anterolateral aspect of the annulus. Smaller arteries and veins, such as the iliolumbar artery and external vertebral veins, can be damaged resulting, at worst, in a retroperitoneal hematoma.

CSF Puncture

It is possible, by taking the vertical approach to the disc space, to enter the foramen and do a subarachnoid puncture. Using an open-bore cannula for the first pass makes this error readily apparent when CSF backflows through the cannula.

Infection

Infection is a potential complication of any invasive surgical procedure. The technical error that may result in the devastating complication of a gram negative discitis is penetration of the bowel during passage of the probe into the disc space. Infection from poor sterile technique will be addressed by other authors in this volume.

Conclusion

Change is part of life in medicine. When properly directed, it is called progress. The lateral approach to the disc space using the intertransverse window of opportunity into the intradiscal interval is presenting new avenues for treatment of lumbar spine disorders. With the pitfalls of chemonucleolysis, and with the realization that the microscope can be used to limit surgical insult to the back, numerous authors, most present at this symposium, have proposed further surgical refinement in the form of percutaneous procedures for lumbar discal pathology. To accomplish this lesser invasive spinal procedure, it is necessary to know the anatomy of the lateral approach. Before anyone condemns percutaneous discectomy by the lateral approach, they should master the technique of lateral discal puncture (Fig. 24).

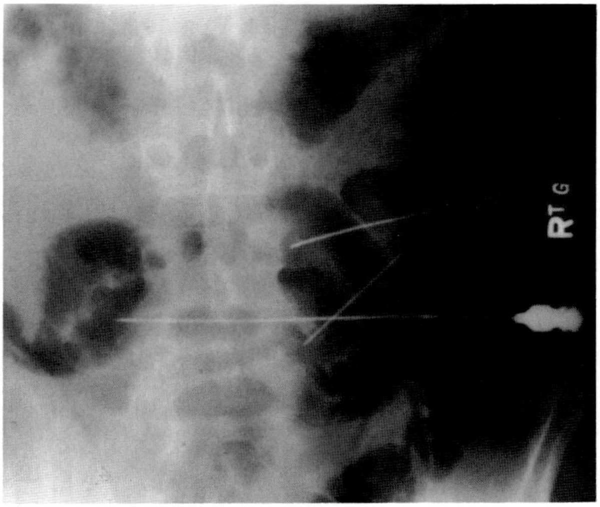

Fig. 24. The surgeon who tried to place these needles in the 3 lower lumbar discs concluded that chemonucleolysis was a useless procedure. He failed to master the technique, yet condemned the procedure. Is that fair?

References

1. Holscher EC (1954) Major vascular complications of intervertebral disc surgery. Ann Surg 140:342–348
2. Kambin P, Myles DB (1987) Percutaneous posterolateral discectomy. Anatomy and mechanism. Clin Orthop 223:145–154
3. Kambin P, Sampson S (1986) Posterolateral percutaneous suction – excision of herniated lumbar intervertebral discs. Clin Orthop 207:37–43
4. Lindblom K (1948) Diagnostic puncture of the intervertebral disc in sciatica. Acta Orthop Scand 17:231–239
5. McCulloch JA, Waddell G (1978) Lateral lumbar discography. Br J Radiol 51:498–502
6. Onik G, Helms C, Ginsberg L, Hoagland T, Morris J (1985) Percutaneous lumbar discectomy using a new aspiration probe. AJNR 6:290–293
7. Schreiber A, Suezawa Y (1986) Transdiscoscopic percutaneous nucleotomy in disc herniation. Orthop Rev 15:75–79
8. Smith L, Brown JE (1967) Treatment of lumbar intervertebral disc lesions by direct injection of chymopapain. J Bone Joint Surg 49B:502–519
9. Yoshizawa H, O'Brien JP, Smith WT et al. (1980) The neuropathology of intervertebral disc removed for low back pain. J Pathol 132:95–104

Intervertebral Disc Material Gained by Percutaneous Discectomy

R. FERSZT [1], S. PATT [2], and H.M. MAYER [3]

Introduction

Considering the vast number of patients operated upon for protruded or herniated lumbar discs, there is comparatively little literature available on the pathology of these structures. One reason for this is that the material gained at surgery is not routinely screened by a pathologist in many neurosurgical centers unless it is of unusual appearance to the surgeon; the rationale being that 1. disc morphology has no immediate clinical relevance, and 2. current in vivo imaging techniques allow early preoperative recognition of lesions other than degenerative disc pathology. Although the latter point is in line with our experience of the past 10 years, surprising pathological findings do occur occasionally, a fact that is well documented in recent literature [4, 5]. Furthermore, Beatty recently suggested the syndrome of myxomatous degeneration, a distinct entity from fibrotic disc degeneration of herniated nucleus pulposus [3]. This condition cannot be diagnosed other than by pathological screening. The popularity of chemonucleolysis has also led to renewed interest in intervertebral disc disease [1].

The aim of this study is to compare the pathological findings in the first 50 cases of percutaneous discectomy performed at the Department of Neurosurgery, Klinikum Steglitz, Freie Universität Berlin, with material gained from a randomized series of lumbar discs resected by conventional techniques.

Material

The group of percutaneous discectomies comprised 50 patients, ages ranging from 12 to 55 years, who had a duration of symptoms ranging from 1 to 15 months and who were operated upon employing the technique described elsewhere in this book (see article by H. M. Mayer and M. Brock). All material was gained either from the intervertebral space L2/L3 or L4/L5. On the average, 5.3 g of material was gained by percutaneous discectomy fixed in 10% formaldehyde embedded in paraffin and stained for H & E, PAS and elastica. The material was evaluated semiquantitatively under the light microscope. As a control group,

[1] Abteilung für Psychiatrie, [2] Institut für Neuropathologie, [3] Abteilung für Neurochirurgie, Klinikum Steglitz, Freie Universität Berlin, Hindenburgdamm 30, 1000 Berlin 45, FRG

Percutaneous Lumbar Discectomy
Ed. by H. M. Mayer and M. Brock

50 samples of material gained by microsurgical interlaminar fenestration from our total series of 700 cases were studied in an identical manner.

The main pathological parameters measured were, the appearance of coarse collagen fibers in the amorphous ground substance in H & E and van Gieson stains ("fibrillation"). Chondrocyte cloning, i.e., the formation of aggregates of chondrocytes, microvacuolar or granular change of the ground substance, myxomatous degeneration, necrosis, tears of the anulus fibrosus, neovascularization of the fibrotic disc tissue, interspersing with fibroblastic proliferation, lymphocellular perivascular infiltrates, as well as signs for traumatization of surrounding tissues such as acute hemorrhages and bone splinters.

Results

The results are given in Table 1, an anatomical view in figures 1–3. There is a clear difference in the spectrum of pathological changes when both groups of patients are compared. Material from the microsurgical series shows a higher density of collagenization in the anulus fibrosus as well as in the nucleus pulposus which is not easily explained by the comparatively slight difference in the average ages (Fig. 4). Furthermore, in individual cases young "open" surgery patients give identical results. The same holds true for microvacuolar or granular change in the ground substance, which is considerably less pronounced in patients with percutaneous discectomy (Fig. 5), even when in individual cases patients of comparable ages are compared. Chondrocyte cloning, considered a regenerative phenomenon

Table 1. Morphological results: Fibrocartilage material microsurgery versus percutaneous discectomy

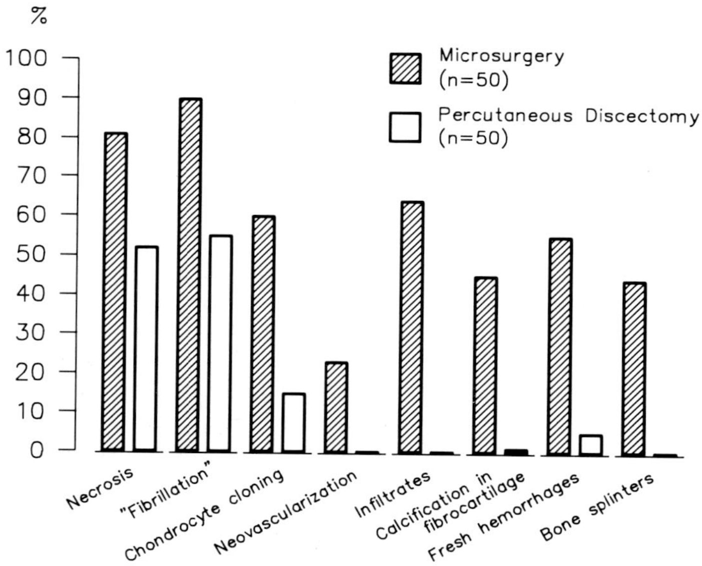

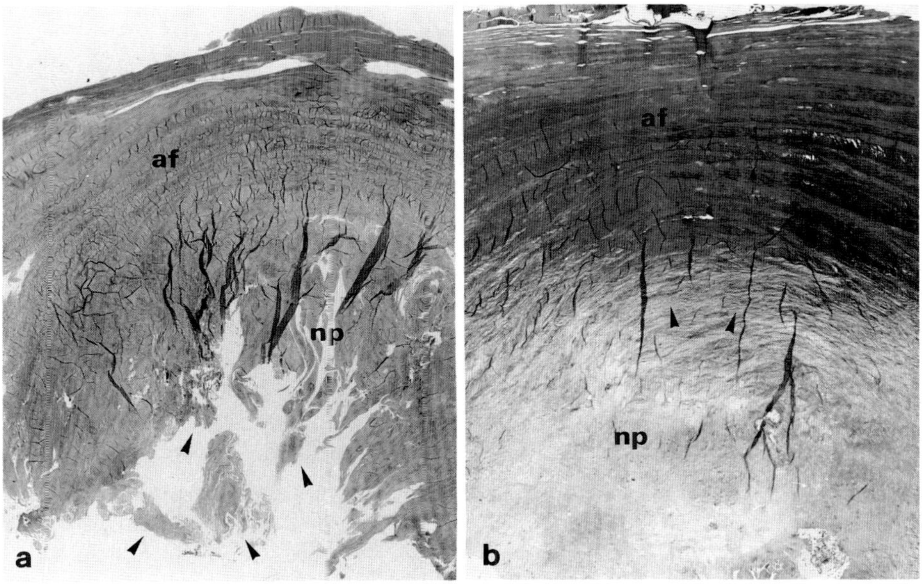

Fig. 1 a, b. The cross-section (elastica van Gieson) of the anulus fibrosus and nucleus pulposus obtained at autopsy (15 ×). **a** 72-year-old patient with severe degenerative disc changes: The border between the nucleus pulposus (*np*) and the anulus fibrosus (*af*) is hard to define because of collagenization and extensive necroses (*arrows*). **b** 30-year-old patient with slight degenerative disc changes: sharply delineated nucleus pulposus (*np*), slight collagenization at borders of nucleus pulposus (*arrows*), no proliferation of chondrocytes, no necroses

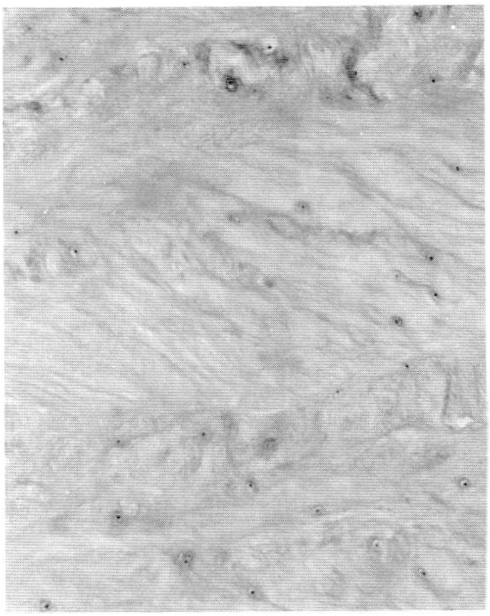

Fig. 2. A higher magnification of the anulus fibrosus (100 ×) with collagen fibers and chondrocytes. The material was taken by percutaneous discectomy and shows practically no degenerative changes

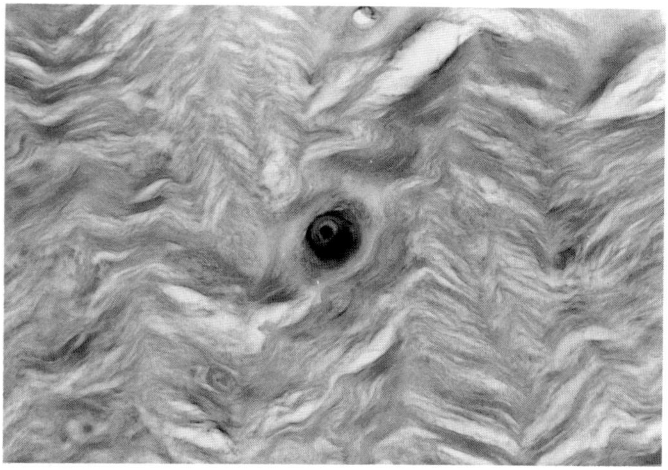

Fig. 3. A higher magnification (400 ×) of the inner border of the anulus fibrosus shows a solitary chondrocyte embedded in masses of horizontally oriented collagen fibers with a typical wavy appearance

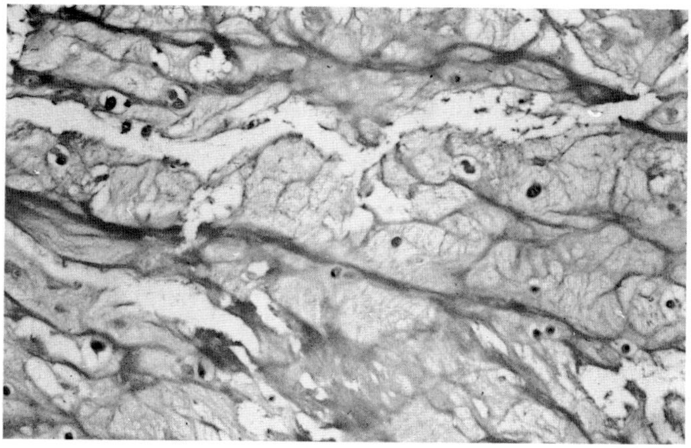

Fig. 4. Visualization of collagen fibers as coarse eosinophilic bands, multiple tears in the fibrocartilage, some necroses (H & E stain, 100 ×)

(Figs. 6, 7), is hardly seen in the percutaneous discectomy group, while it is a regular finding in the control series (Fig. 8). Myxomatous change as defined by Beatty was not seen in our total series of 100 cases. Neovascularization (Fig. 9) was seen in about 15% of the "open" surgery patients, but never in the percutaneous discectomy group. Identical findings were made as far as infiltrates are concerned (Figs. 9, 10). Necroses were often demonstrable in microsurgical material (Figs. 11, 12). In percutaneous biopsies, there were only occasional small, fresh, necrotic areas.

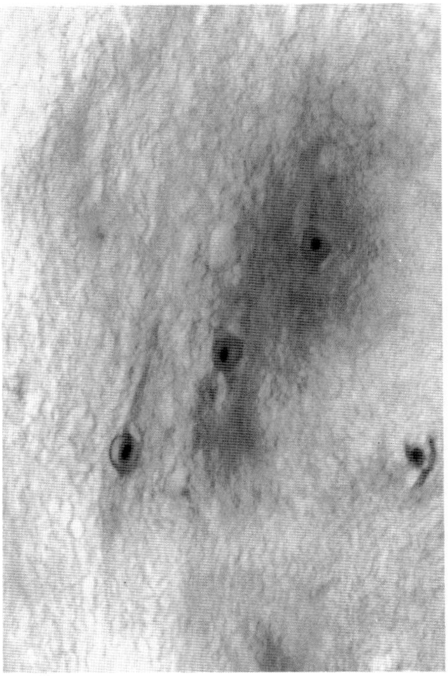

Fig. 5. Material from percutaneous discectomy (400 ×): Only a few normal sized chondrocytes are visible. The ground substance is intact

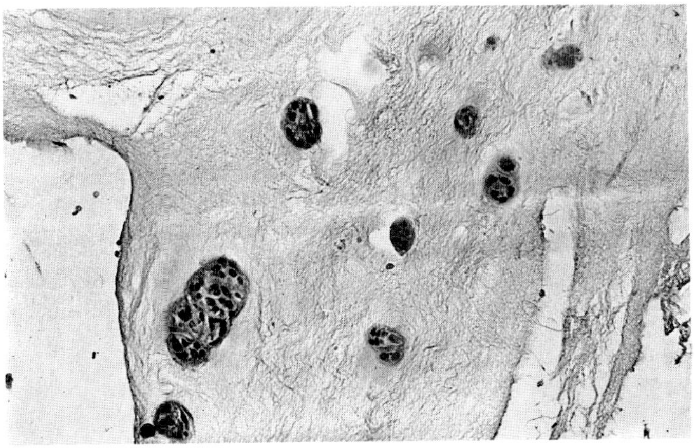

Fig. 6. Low-power magnification (40 ×) of "chondrocyte cloning" in cartilage also showing microvacuolar or granular degeneration

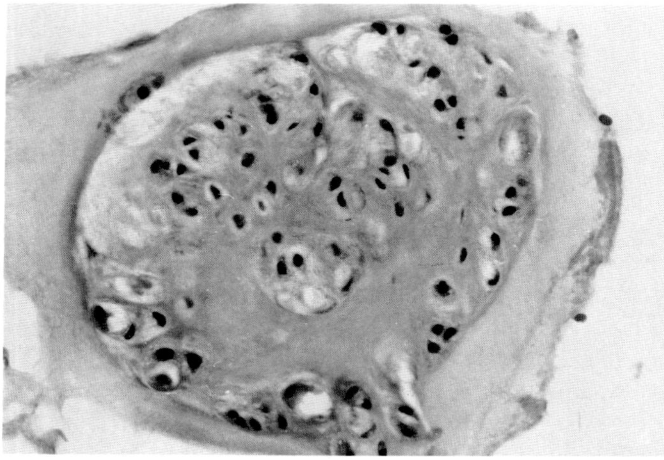

Fig. 7. High power (400 ×) magnification of an aggregate of chondrocytes typically seen in severe degenerative disc disease

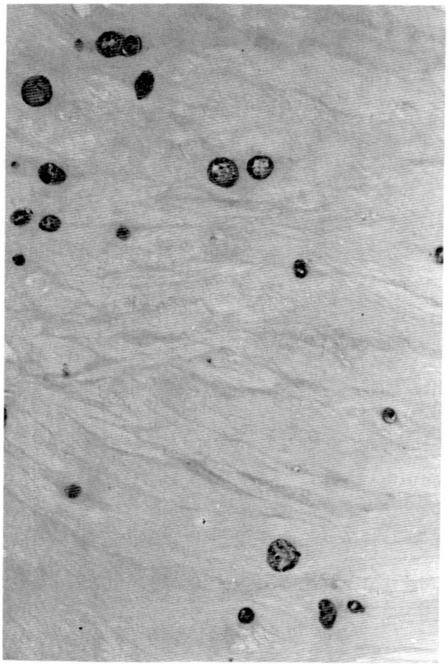

Fig. 8

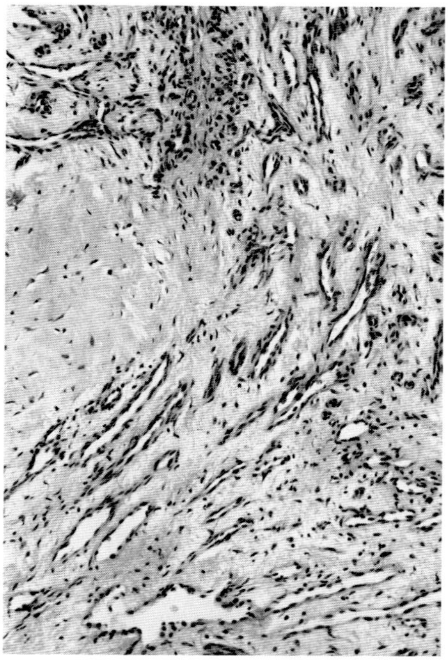

Fig. 9

Fig. 8. Chondrocyte cloning with marked fibrosis at the border of the nucleus pulposus (H & E stain, 40 ×)

Fig. 9. Extensive neovascularization of herniated fibrocartilage; mostly capillaries and venules are involved, many of them show lymphocellular infiltrates. This picture is typical of subacute disc prolapse

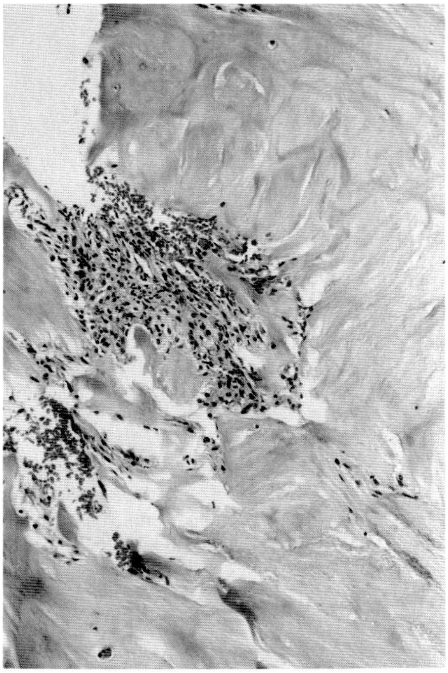

Fig. 10. Collagen fibers in fibrocartilage, reactive fibroplasia and pericapillary lymphocellular infiltrates, some fresh hemorrhage in a case of longstanding disc prolapse

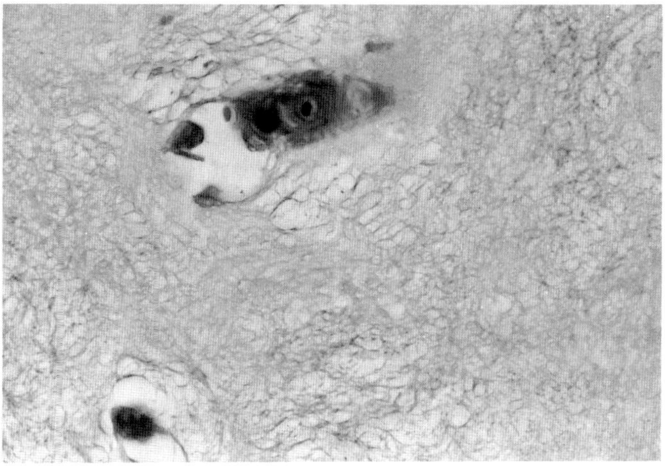

Fig. 11. Necrotic cartilage surrounding a partly calcified chondrocyte. The ground substance is hardly stained and shows some vacuolar degeneration (H & E stain, 100×)

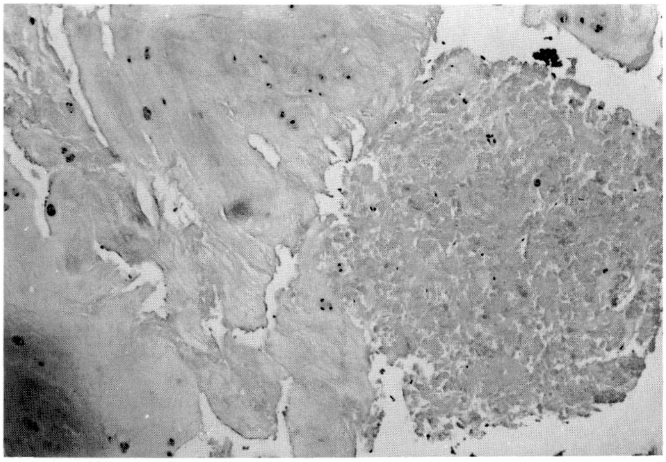

Fig. 12. Necrosis of fibrocartilage in herniated disc; the tissue at the right side of the picture has lost its texture and consists mainly of loosely arranged debris with some cell remnants. The remaining fibrocartilage shows marked degeneration

Discussion

Our results indicate that patients undergoing percutaneous discectomy are a group distinct from those operated upon by more conventional techniques. This is not due to their slightly lower average age, but to the fact that their discs have a typical pathology.

Peripheral neovascularization of the anulus fibrosus may in our experience be considered a reliable indicator for prolapsed intervertebral disc material. This fits in with the recent paper by Weidner and Rice who in 1988 revealed the histological features of curetted fibrocartilage from 100 consecutive patients at Harvard Medical School [9]. While the fact that neovascularization has occurred in the fibrocartilage reliably indicates prolapse, the degree of lymphocellular reaction may vary considerably. As yet, we have not been able to corroborate the latter with clinical parameters. Both features were absent in the percutaneous discectomy series.

The tissue sample gained by the percutaneous route is much smaller than that resected by microsurgery, but, this does not change the trend in our data; according to Aufdermaur 1984, Lyons et al. 1966, Sokoloff 1969, and Naylor et al. 1975, prolapsed nucleus pulposus tissue shows maximal degenerative changes in intervertebral disc material. As the resection of the protruded pulposus is the aim of the percutaneous technique, it is probable that the tissue gained by this route represents maximal degenerative changes in that disc.

Judging from our results, patients undergoing percutaneous discectomy, regardless of the duration of symptoms, belong to a group with less pronounced degenerative disc disease than those treated microsurgically.

Further studies are warranted to assess whether successful percutaneous discectomy will be limited to this group of patients or whether it is applicable to the prolapsed and more severely degenerated intervertebral disc.

References

1. Artigas J, Brock M, Mayer HM (1984) Complications following chemonucleolysis with collagenase. J Neurosurg 61:679–685
2. Aufdermaur M (1984) Bandscheibendegenerationen und ihre Folgen. In: Doerr W, Seifert G (Hrsg) Pathologie der Gelenke und Weichteiltumoren, Bd 18 II. Springer, Berlin Heidelberg New York Tokyo, S 1074–1086
3. Beatty RA (1985) Myxomatous degeneration of the lumbar intervertebral disc. Neurosurgery 17:277–280
4. Bergemer AM, Fouquet B, Goupille P, Born P, Cosnay P, Fauchier JP, Valat JP (1987) Intervertebral disc space infections revealing acute bacterial endocarditis. A report of 4 cases and a review of the literature. Rhumatologie 39:195–199
5. Kala M, Chrobok J, Dvorak P (1987) A surprising finding by a surgery for lumbar intervertebral disk herniation, Ewing's sarcoma. Acta Univ Polacki Olomuc Fac Med 117:185–189
6. Lyons H, Jones E, Quinn FE, Sprunt DH (1966) Changes in the protein-polysaccharide fractions of nucleus pulposus from human intervertebral disc with age and disc degeneration. J Lab Clin Med 68:930–939
7. Naylor A, Happey F, Turner RL, Shentall RD, West DC, Richardson C (1975) Enzymic and immunological activity in the intervertebral disc. Orthop Clin North Am 6:51–58
8. Sokoloff L (1969) The biology of degenerative joint disease. University of Chicago Press, Chicago, London
9. Weidner N, Rice DT (1988) Intervertebral disk material: criteria for determining probable prolapse. Hum Pathol 19:406–410

Pathophysiology

Biomechanical Background of Low Back Pain, Sciatica and Flexion Therapy

J. KRÄMER and W. KUEHNEGGER [1]

Most patients with chronic low back problems experience pain relief when they flatten their lumbar lordosis by flexion of knees and hips. Our patients learn this in the Back School.

In the myelogram we can see a flattening of a bulging disc by forward bending.

Not all back problems do result from disc protrusions. The majority of patients with low back pain only have degenerative instability of their motion segments. During disc degeneration the motion segments loose stability and height. Combined with a weakness of the abdominal muscles the lower lumbar segments are compressed in a lordotic position during lifting of heavy goods or even just by standing in an upright position.

With axial loading of lumbar segments a telescopic longitudinal movement of the articular facets takes place.

This increases if loading is combined with lordosis and if the segment has lost stability by degeneration, trauma, discectomy, chemonucleolysis or percutaneous discectomy.

In an unstable lumbar motion segment in most cases pain comes from the posterior longitudinal ligament and the vertebral joint capsules, which are known to have many pressure and tension-sensitive nerve endings.

Table 1. Experiments in the Dept. for Biomechanics, Orthop. Univ. Bochum

1. Volume-changes of the spinal canal by fluid and plastic fillings [2]
2. Volume-changes of the vertebral joints [4]
3. Tension of the longitudinal ligaments by using mercury strain gages [1]
4. Tension of the vertebral joint capsules using mercury strain gages [1]
5. Registration of the center of rotation by photometry

On the other hand hyperlordosis of the lumbar spine can provoke nerve root compression in the intervertebral foramen and spinal stenosis symptoms.

In our bioengineering department for functional morphologic anatomy we performed several experiments to record all changes in the motion segment which develop by degenerative disc instability and movements, such as flexion extension, lateral bending and torsion (Table 1 and 2).

[1] Orthopädische Universitätsklinik, St. Josefs-Hospital, Gudrunstr. 56, 4630 Bochum, FRG

Percutaneous Lumbar Discectomy
Ed. by H. M. Mayer and M. Brock

Table 2. Loading an unstable lumbar motion segment leads to following changes:

1. Bulging of the anulus and posterior longitudinal ligament
2. Reduction of the spinal canal volume
3. Narrowing of the intervertebral foramen
4. Facet joints are moved telescopically
5. Facet joint capsules are stretched
6. Center of rotation moves backwards

Details about our experiments of volume changes have already been published [4]. In our recent experiments about length and tension changes in longitudinal ligaments and facet joint capsules of lumbar motion segments under various conditions we measured flexibility in all directions under load with and without experimental instability. Motion segment instability was achieved by denucleation of the disc which can be compared with the behavior of degenerated discs [5].

Material and Methods

Lumbar motion segments were fixed into a special frame which allowed movements in all directions under physiological load (flexion, extension, side bending, rotation).

Mercury-in-rubber strain gages (MSG) were fixed to the longitudinal ligaments and to the joint capsules following the fiber directions. They measured changes in length of these structures. Stretching the MSG leads to a reduction in the cross sectional area and to an increase in length of the mercury filament, resulting in an increase of electrical resistance.

The specimens were brought into different positions under load before and after removal of the nucleus in order to simulate degenerative instability.

In flexion, extension, lateral bending, torsion and in combined movements there is a certain tension in the posterior longitudinal ligament and in different parts of the joint capsule.

In an unstable segment, after removal of the nucleus, tension of the posterior longitudinal ligament and in the joint capsule is higher than in a normal segment. Slight flexion of about 8 degrees normalizes the tension of the posterior longitudinal ligament and the joint capsule. We call this the relaxation point. Relaxation of the joint capsules persists even if additional lateral bending takes place.

Other kinds of movements, such as further flexion, extension and lateral bending, cause an increase of tension in all ligaments and joint capsule structures. The angle of maximum relaxation in a loaded degenerative segment results from the fact that downward motion of the inferior articular process begins to stretch the upper capsule at a certain point. In the first stage of flexion the ends of the ligaments get closer together which leads to a relaxation of the joint capsule. Flexion above the point of relaxation stretches the capsule again (Table 3).

Table 3. Slight flexion of a loaded unstable lumbar motion segment leads to following changes:

1. The previously bulged anulus and posterior longitudinal ligament are straightened, tension is normalized
2. Enlargement of the spinal canal volume
3. Enlargement of the intervertebral foramen
4. Position of the facet joints is normalized
5. Facet joint capsule is relaxed
6. Center of rotation moves into its previous central position

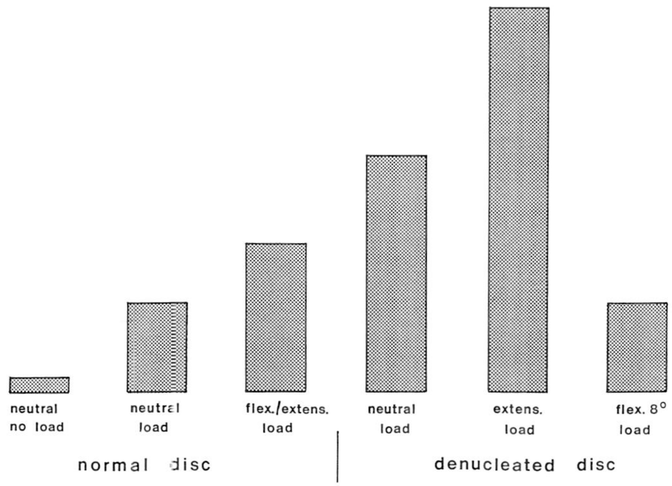

Fig. 1. Tension in the lumbar vertebral joint capsules after loading a normal and a denucleated disc

Conclusion

In a degenerated unstable motion segment with a reduced disc height the posterior longitudinal ligament and the vertebral joint capsules are already stretched in the mid-position when the segment is loaded. People suffer from low back pain when they are standing. This pain increases when extension with hyperlordosis takes place.

Slight flexion up to the relaxation point brings pain relief. In our Back School the patients can reach this relaxation point by bending their knees and hips in order to flatten their lumbar lordosis.

Abdominal muscle training and training of the pelvic tilt lead to a flattening of the lumbar lordosis.

In order to relieve pain, patients are brought into the ninety-ninety position (flexion of ninety degrees for hips and knees). In this position they can also do their abdominal muscle training without pain.

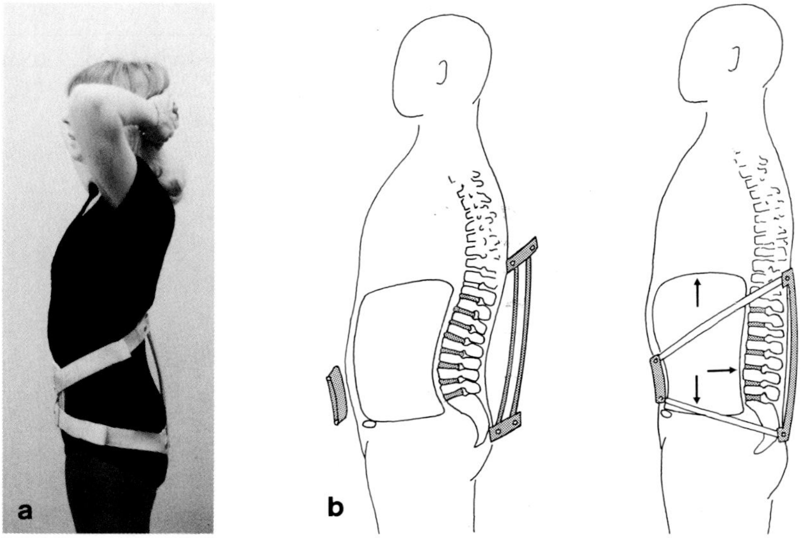

Fig. 2a, b. Flexion orthosis lumboflex. The suprapubically located abdominal pad connected to the bridging lumbosacral support produces a 3-point system which reduces the lumbar lordosis by flexion. The dynamic design feature permits body motion in all except the lordotic direction

Table 4. Flexion therapy

1. Flattening of the lumbar curve in back school; pelvic tilt, back straight
2. Abdominal muscle training
3. Ninety-ninety position
4. Flexion orthosis – lumboflex
5. Lumbo Sacral Distraction Spondylodesis (LSDS)

In our bioengineering department we developed a dynamic flexion brace (Lumboflex) which allows all kinds of movements except extension (Fig. 2).

Facet infiltration with local anaesthetics give relief to the overstretched joint capsules, especially if the infiltration is followed by flexion exercises.

The last stage of flexion therapy is the lumbosacral distraction spondylodesis, which keeps up the flexion point.

We are currently working on a flexion program also for the cervical spine syndrome, because there are almost the same problems of ligamentous overstretching by hyperlordosis (Table 4).

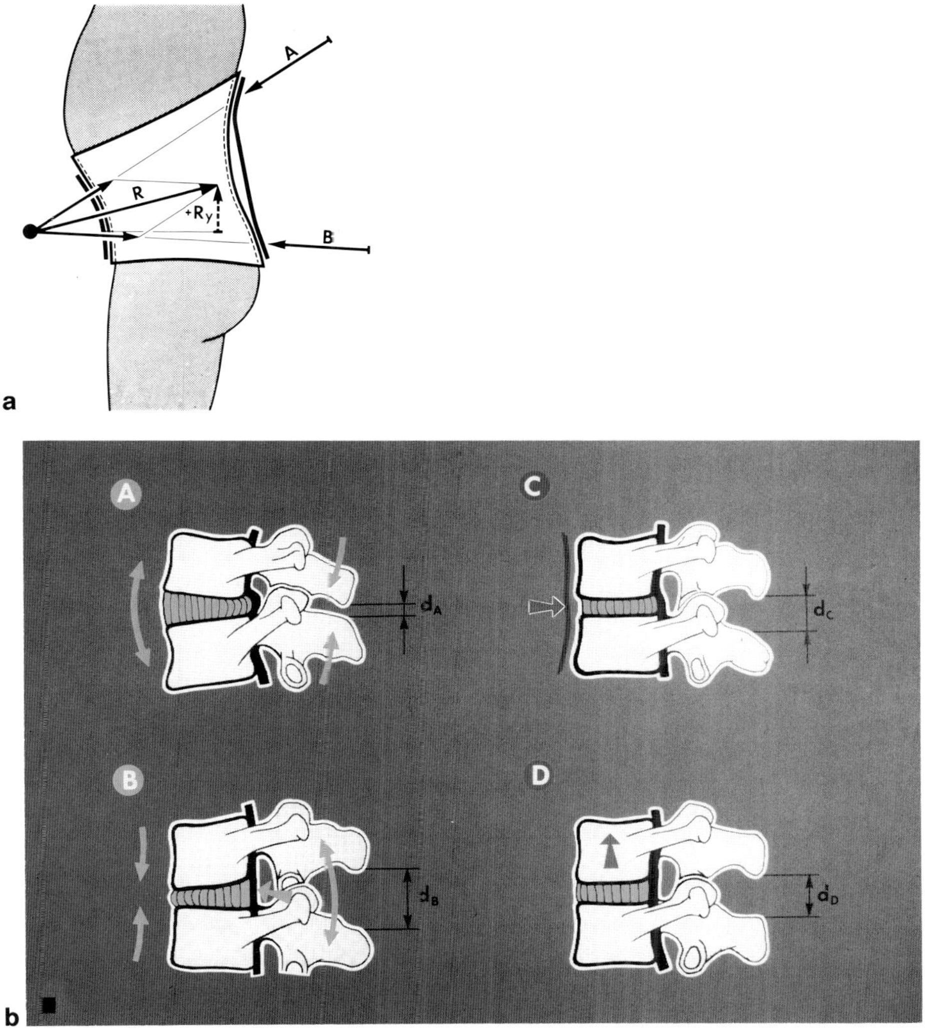

Fig. 3a, b. Dynamic flexion therapy is achieved by the 3-point system. **a** Direct mechanical tension straps produce the resultant force *R* as intraabdominal pressure with a cranially directed force vector + Ry for direct unloading of the lumbar spine. **b** The bending moment produced by the forces *A* and *B* reduces the hyperlordosis in the lumbosacral region and realigns the intervertebral positions.

The dynamic design principle inherent in the material selection of the components permits body motion in all except the lordotic direction.

The patient is thus not totally immobilized but restrained selectively in the critical position without undue atrophic side effects

References

1. Hedtmann A, Steffen R, Methfessel J, Kolditz D, Krämer J, Thols M (1989) Measurement of human lumbar spine ligaments during loaded and unloaded motion. Spine 14:175–185
2. Krämer J (1981) Intervertebral disc diseases. Thieme Inc, New York
3. Krämer J (1986) Bandscheibenbedingte Erkrankungen, 2. Aufl. Thieme, Stuttgart
4. Krämer J, Kaschner A (1981) Zur Biomechanik der Wirbelgelenke an der Lendenwirbelsäule. In: Junghanns H (Hrsg) Die Wirbelsäule in Forschung und Praxis 87:149
5. Krag MH, Seroussi RE, Muller D, Pope MH (1987) Effect of denucleation on the internal deformations of the intervertebral disc. Abstracts ISSLS, Rome 1987

Diagnosis

The Clinical Diagnosis of Lumbar Disc Disease

P. MARX [1]

Lecturing on the clinical diagnosis of lumbar disc disease is a difficult task. Since every one of you is experienced in this field, it seems to me that I am carrying coal to Newcastle, so to speak. On the other hand, the role of a neurologist has changed somewhat from the days of Gowers, who asked Alexander Horsley to operate on a tumor that he diagnosed clinically without the aid of technical methods. Nowadays the neurologist often gets the impression that patients are being operated upon for disc disease diagnosed by imaging procedures that might have benefited more from conservative measures. Sometimes we are even faced with the fact that a patient has been operated on for a disc prolapse that was completely unrelated to his complaints. Thus it might be of interest to delineate the diagnostic strategies a neurologist uses to choose the best treatment for a given patient.

In a case history, one must not only get a clear description of pain, muscle weakness, and bladder function, but also of present and past diseases and complaints. Since pain perception is strongly modulated by limbic influences, information about the patient's psychosocial background is of utmost importance. I would just like to remind you of the so-called "young executive syndrome" and the many depressive patients who complain about backache or sciatica who would benefit more from antidepressants than from surgical treatment, even if disc protrusion or herniation is present. Unfortunately, time does not allow me to go into the further details of this extremely important aspect of patient examination.

Looking through textbooks on orthopedics and neuroorthopedics, it is obvious that much emphasis is being placed on inspection, palpation, and functional testing of the lumbar spine, the sacro-iliacal joints, and the hip joints. The patient's posture and movement admittedly do give many clues to the location of the underlying disease, and functional testing and palpation may be an even better means of determining the site of a lesion. Most, if not all, of these parameters are unspecific, however, and require additional sources of information.

This can be exemplified by the straight-leg raising test, called Lasègue's sign, which is considered indicative of disc herniation. Lasègue's sign is indeed positive in most patients with root compression syndromes at levels L 5 or S 1, but not at higher levels, where the femoral stretch test becomes positive instead. However,

[1] Neurologische Klinik und Poliklinik, Klinikum Steglitz, Freie Universität Berlin, Hindenburgdamm 30, 1000 Berlin 45, FRG

Percutaneous Lumbar Discectomy
Ed. by H. M. Mayer and M. Brock

Lasègue's sign may also be positive in other conditions such as polyneuropathy, lyme disease radiculitis, and meningiosis carcinomatosa, to name a few.

In some cases of L 5 compression, Lasègue's sign may be absent, even in the presence of major neurological dysfunctions. In my personal experience, a root compression syndrome which is mainly motor and only rarely sensory where this sign is negative is indicative of a foraminal prolapse, which will not respond to conservative treatment. One should therefore recommend early surgery for these patients and avoid useless time delay with conservative treatments.

It is my opinion that, as long as Lasègue's and other known vertebral signs are positive, the chances for successful conservative treatment are much better.

I cannot imagine why many orthopedic textbooks recommend that neurological examinations be done only in selected cases. Since lower back pain and/or sciatica may be caused by various neurological diseases, a thorough examination is mandatory *in every case*. This examination must give information on the condition of cranial nerves as well as the motor, sensory, and vegetative systems. In lumbar spine disease, detailed single-muscle function testing in the lower extremities is mandatory. Bilateral tendon reflex comparisons, Babinski's sign, and other indicators of spasticity, bladder and bowel function, and, last but not least, sensory irritations or defects should also be investigated.

I would like to point out the fact that lumbar disc herniation very often involves the anterior root, thus causing corresponding muscular paresis without sensory loss. Since the muscular nerve supply is organized in myotomes, each anterior root supplies only a few specific muscles. In almost all cases, analysis of the pattern of muscle dysfunction therefore allows exact identification of the root involved.

In an S 1 lesion, the short peroneal muscle, the gastrocnemius muscle, and the biceps femoris may be affected. Accordingly, the patient may experience weakness of foot pronation and have difficulties standing on the tips of his toes. If the paresis is only slight, it can be diagnosed by comparison with the contralateral side. Concomitantly, the Achilles tendon reflex is diminished or even absent as compared with the contralateral side, and this sign is often the only remnant of an old S 1 involvement.

The specific muscle of L 5 is the extensor hallucis longus, and a paresis of this muscle is very often the only objective sign of this very common root compression syndrome. Foot elevation and, especially, pronation (peroneus longus and brevis) may sometimes also be affected as hip abduction. Severe paresis of the anterior tibial muscle is, however, not characteristic of an L 5 compression syndrome. Patellar and Achilles tendon reflexes are normal in uncomplicated cases of L 5 syndrome, but the Achilles tendon reflex may be diminished or absent when there is an accompanying S 1 lesion. In an L 5 lesion, the reflex of the tibialis posterior muscle is usually absent, but since it is normally a very weak and inconstant reflex, this sign is relevant only if the reflex on the contralateral side is normal.

Compression of the L 4 root leads to paresis of the anterior tibial muscle. Slight weakness of the quadriceps femoris muscle becomes evident when the patient steps up on a chair. The patellar tendon reflex is diminished or absent.

An L 3 lesion is characterized by severe dysfunction of the quadriceps femoris and also involves the adductors. Accordingly, the patellar tendon reflex and the adductor reflexes are absent or diminished. The involvement of the adductors and their reflex allows the neurologist to easily distinguish an L 3 lesion from a femoral nerve lesion.

The supply areas of single dorsal roots are well known by all neurologists, and will not be dealt with in detail here. It might be helpful to repeat that, in many cases, sensory loss has not occurred, and therefore a test of sensory functions is very often less informative in lumbar disc disease than single muscle function tests. However, since pain radiates along the same line, the exact localization of pain may give information about the site of the lesion.

Bladder and bowel function are of particular interest in the clinical diagnosis of lumbar disc disease. The patient therefore must be asked about his ability to micturate. When dysfunction is suspected, the bladder must at least be palpated and the tone of the sphincter ani and the cutaneous anal reflexes must be checked.

Time does not allow me to fully describe the various conditions that should be considered in differential diagnosis of lumbar disc disease. However, I shall discuss some major differences between root dysfunctions and peripheral nerve disease. In rare instances, an S 1 lesion must be distinguished from a tibial nerve disturbance. Differentiation is usually easy: direction of pain radiation, sensory loss if present, and involvement of the biceps femoris and/or the hip abductors rule out a tibial nerve lesion. Additionally sweat secretion on the sole of the foot and on the toes is normal in root compression syndrome, but absent in peripheral nerve disease.

In single-root L 5 compression, separate paresis of the long extensor muscle of the big toe is so characteristic that it is almost impossible to mistake it for any other condition. However, a combined L 5/S 1 lesion sometimes must be distinguished from a peroneal nerve lesion and/or an iatrogenic lesion of the sciatic nerve by false drug injection, which usually involves the peroneal part of this nerve much more than the tibial nerve. Careful documentation of case history, involvement of hip abductors, a combination of a severe paresis of the two short extensors and the foot pronators, yet only mild paresis of the anterior tibial muscle, different sensory loss patterns, and preserved sweat secretion in the supply area of the peroneal nerve point to root compression syndrome. Of course, the Achilles tendon reflex is positive with peroneal nerve lesions, but it may be absent in root compression syndrome as well as in lesions of the sciatic nerve. It is seldom necessary to measure the nerve conduction velocity of the peroneal nerve by electrophysiological means.

Combined L 4/L 5 lesions might be mistaken for peroneal dysfunction or tibialis anterior syndrome. Difficulty in stretching the knee and diminuation or absence of the patellar tendon reflex facilitate differentiation, however. An L 3 lesion can easily be mistaken for femoral nerve disease. Clinical differentiation is easy if one looks for involvement of the adductors and their reflexes, which are disturbed in root compression syndrome, but not in femoral nerve dysfunction. Additionally, sensory disturbances, if present, vary greatly in the two conditions.

These very few examples are intended to demonstrate the fact that the neurological examination almost always allows exact clinical identification of the nervous structures involved, be it in the root or the peripheral nerve. At this point, I would like to make a very fundamental statement. Although the neurological examination can tell us where the lesion or irritation is, it will never be able to tell us with certainty what the etiology of the syndrome is. Empirically, an L 5 syndrome caused by the disc herniation is not different from an L 5 compression caused by a tumor. Etiological differentiation is possible only with the aid of additional information on case history, concomitant physical abnormalities and, in particular, data from imaging techniques and laboratory testing.

Here, again, the importance of the neurological examination becomes evident. Very often, the patient presents to the neurologist CT scans or even myelograms that have been taken at the wrong spinal level or in cases with polyneuropathy, i.e. in cases with peripheral nervous diseases. This situation becomes particularly dangerous for the patient if an unrelated and clinically innocent disc herniation is spotted and subjected to useless surgery.

Since Trittmacher and Purmann will be handling the neuroradiological diagnosis of lumbar disc disease, I shall not touch upon this topic directly. I would just like to briefly mention that in every case in which a myelography is performed, a CSF sample of about 5 cc should be drawn before any dye is injected into the spine. Cell count and cell and protein differentiation tests should be performed. A spinal tap does not increase the incidence of postlumbar puncture syndrome, but it may very often give valuable additional information. This is particularly the case in ill-indicated myelographies, which occur, for instance, when root irritation syndrome is caused by multiple sclerosis, lyme disease radiculitis, or meningeosis carcinomatosa. After dye has been injected, the CSF is altered for many weeks, which makes correct diagnosis extremely difficult or even impossible.

I would also like to mention that even large disc herniations demonstrated by CT or myelography may leave the patient absolutely free of symptoms. Root irritation syndromes might be caused by radiculitis, despite concomitant disc herniation. Thus a radiographically diagnosed disc disease is only relevant if it matches the clinical syndrome.

In conclusion, it can be said that no single investigation, be it orthopedic, neurologic, radiologic, MRI or laboratory, can by itself constitute a valid diagnosis of a lumbar spine disease. Only if all available information fits together can the diagnosis be considered safe. A thorough neurological examination is an integral part of this combined investigation, and it should be performed in every patient.

Radiodiagnostics of the Lumbar Spine

S. TRITTMACHER and H. PURMANN[1]

Many imaging techniques have been applied to the lumbar vertebral column. The most important among the current radiologic examinations are:

- plain X-ray of the spine
- discography
- myelography
- CT and myelo-CT
- MRI

In the following, we will briefly review some salient aspects of these procedures and will especially stress their advantages and shortcomings.

Plain X-ray

Alterations in the vertebral column and its soft tissues due to disc degeneration can be seen on standard plain films [2]. The most frequent signs are:

- narrowing of the disk interspaces
- increased density of the vertebral end plates
- soft tissue calcification

Furthermore, there might be dorsal displacement of the vertebra, scoliosis and a decrease or total loss of lumbar lordosis. However, these indirect signs are not specific for disc herniation and are therefore of limited value. The main task of plain films is, therefore, to rule out any other pathology, such as:

- malformation
- neoplasia
- osteoporosis
- spondylolisthesis
- spondylitis
- Paget's disease

[1] Klinik für Diagnostische Radiologie und Nuklearmedizin, Klinikum Steglitz, Freie Universität Berlin, Hindenburgdamm 30, 1000 Berlin 45, FRG

Percutaneous Lumbar Discectomy
Ed. by H. M. Mayer and M. Brock

Discography

For discography, a needle is introduced into the central portion of the disk, and a small amount of contrast medium is injected. This procedure can be performed under fluoroscopy or CT guidance. Normally, the contrast medium pools centrally in the nucleus pulposus. In degenerated discs, the contrast medium forms a more irregular shape and diffuses into more peripheral parts of the disc. In view of the possible side effects and given the availability of CT and MRI, discography has lost its importance and is performed very seldom today [2].

Myelography

Imaging of neural tissues within the spinal canal remained elusive in the abovementioned techniques and led to the idea of opacification of subarachnoid space. With the development of water-soluble contrast medium, the number of myelograms increased enormously. Still, in the early eighties, myelography was the method of choice in evaluation of lumbar disc herniation [1, 2].

Disc herniation is manifested on a myelogram as a filling defect and a displacement of the dural sac and nerve root pouches. Its contour can be flat, curved, or nearly round. When seen in profile, the margins are always sharply defined. The extent of the filling defect varies from flat depression, through an increasingly deep indentation to a complete stop of contrast passage.

The most important feature for evaluation of the root pouches is the comparison to the opposite side. Compression of a nerve root is manifested as a break in the usual linear, slightly curved image of the root which often widens above its entry into the root canal.

Compression of root pouches results in decreased filling with contrast medium. With complete filling defects, the pouches are simply not seen. When filling is partial, the medial, lateral, or distal portion may be missing. "Shortening" or "amputation" of the root pouch is the most common and most important finding (Fig. 1).

It is not always easy to differentiate between a prolapse and a protrusion, since the important structures (anulus fibr., post. long. lig.) cannot be directly imaged. If ventral impression of the epidural space above or below the affected disc compartment is shown and there is no evidence of contact with the disc, then one can conclude that there might be a sequestered disc herniation. But in case the myelogram appears normal at first glance, one certainly should take additional pictures with the patient in the upright position, in reclination, and anteclination. If the compression of the dural sac increases under exertion, there is a so-called "soft disc protrusion", where the fibrous ring is still intact (Fig. 2). This is, in our opinion, a great advantage of myelography compared to all other methods, because it allows imaging under daily-life and dynamic conditions.

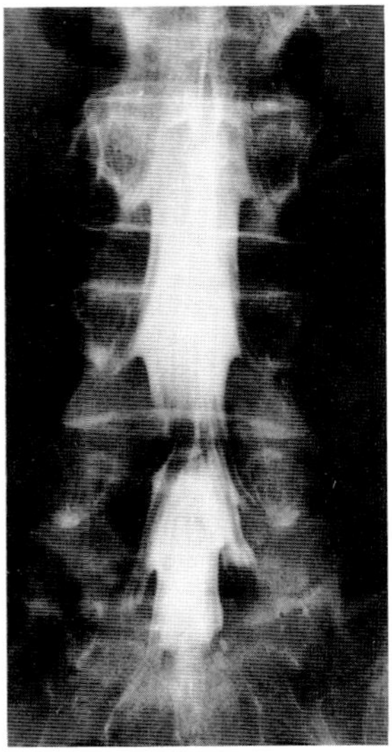

Fig. 1

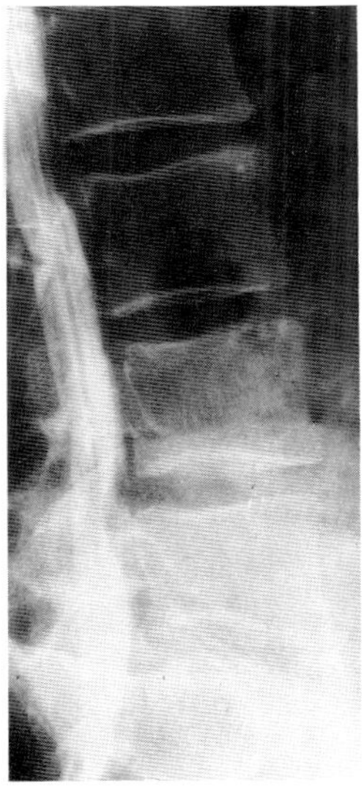

Fig. 2

Fig. 1. Lumbar myelogram, ap-projection: Amputation of L_5-nerve root pouch and compression of adjacent nerve root S_1 due to medio-lateral disc herniation $L_{4/5}$

Fig. 2. Lumbar myelogram, lateral projection: Increased compression of the dural sac with the patient in the upright position and in reclination. (The first series showed a normal myelogram)

High Resolution CT

Due to high contrast resolution, high signal-to-noise ratio, thin slices with little partial volume effects, and short scan times with reduction of motion artefacts, CT scanning of the vertebral column has meanwhile become one of the most often performed examinations in computed tomography practice [1]. The simplest type of spinal CT is the plain examination. It primarily shows bony structures, but also the soft tissues. The contents of the vertebral canal often elude differential evaluation in the plain scan. The entire subarachnoid space is contrasted when the contrast medium is applied intrathecally [1].

Pathological findings are indicated in plain CT as well as contrast CT by displacement or compression and constriction of the dural sac, although fine tissue differences between the nucleus pulposus, the fibrous ring, and the posterior longitudinal ligament cannot be determined.

Protrusions of the disc are diagnosible in plain CT as well as after intrathecal application of contrast medium. An early sign of a degenerative change in disc tissue is the loss of concavity in the dorsal disc borders. A healthy intervertebral disc ends with the border of the vertebra, and only in the segment L 5/S 1 may a protrusion be physiological when there are no further signs of compression. Filling of the lateral recess is in any case pathological, as is flattening of the dural sac (Fig. 3).

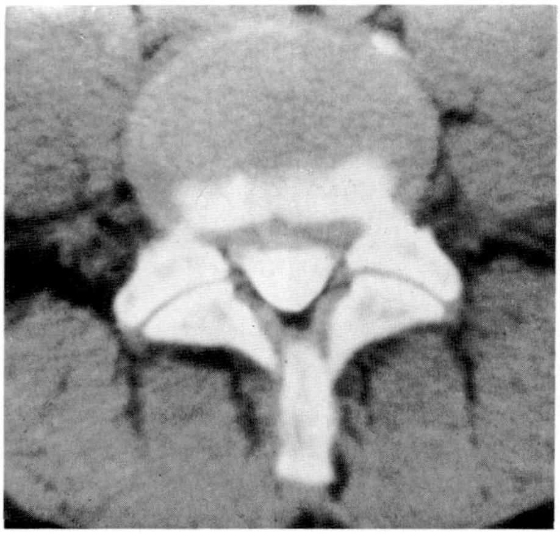

Fig. 3. Spinal computed assisted tomogram. Protrusion of disc tissue. Compression of the dural sac and filling of the lateral recesses. (Subarachnoid space opacified after intrathecal contrast application)

It is noteworthy that, because CT depicts a vertebral column that is at rest, false negative findings can be established. Now and then we have observed this discrepancy in findings obtained by CT and myelography.

MRI

The development of multislice spin-echo pulse sequences, higher magnetic field strength, steeper gradients and special surface coils made MRI superior to all other imaging modalities. One of the advantages of MRI is the free choice of planes [1, 3].

T1-weighted (TR 600–100 ms, TE 2 ms) images provide the best anatomic detail. On midsagittal views, the low-signal cortical bone frames the vertebral body. The nucleus is mid-range in signal intensity, similar to that of nerve roots. The anulus and ligaments are of very low intensity and cannot be distinguished from each other, nor from adjacent cortical bone.

T2-weighted (TR 2000 ms, TE 50/70 ms) images show differences in disc hydration. In aged or desiccated discs, nucleus pulposus and anulus fibrosus can no longer be distinguished, and in completely desiccated discs it is usually not possible to differentiate between disc, osteophyte and cortical bone.

In well hydrated intervertebral discs, the protruding disc tissue can be well delimited from its low signal surroundings, and a definitive statement on the condition of the posterior longitudinal ligament can be made; a rupture is then confirmable (Fig. 4).

Extremely lateral disc herniations located in the foramen are very difficult to diagnose by MRI, because the detail resolution is not yet sufficient.

A further disadvantage is that MRI also depicts the spinal column at rest. Exercise and function tests, which may be of decisive importance in distinguishing between prolapse or protrusion, cannot be performed with MRI.

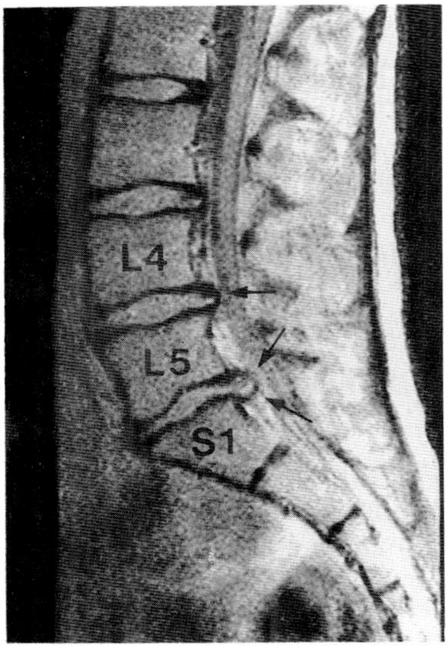

Fig. 4. MRI, midsagittal plane: In case of well hydrated discs the disc herniation is delimited from its low signal surroundings

Since the introduction of water-soluble contrast agents approximately 15 years ago, the importance given to certain special techniques in evaluation of lumbar disk disease has constantly changed. The vertebral canal and its contents comprise a longitudinally oriented system. We therefore prefer longitudinal imaging systems like MRI and myelography. Cross-sectional representation (CT, MRI) can later give specific and essential additional information.

The difficulty of all the techniques described above is how to decide whether a protrusion or prolapse is present, because, up to now, it has not been possible to image the most important structures themselves. The fibrous ring and the posterior longitudenal ligament are identified only as a negative contrast to their surroundings.

In our opinion, MRI will solve this problem in the future.

References

1. Gonzalez C, Grossmann Ch, Masden J (1985) Head and spine imaging. Wiley, New York Chichester Brisbane Toronto Singapore
2. Kautzky R, Zülch K, Wende S, Tänzer A (1976) Neuroradiologie auf neuropathologischer Grundlage. Springer, Berlin Heidelberg New York
3. Lissner J, Seiderer M (1987) Klinische Kernspintomographie. Enke, Stuttgart

Discography and Postdiscographic CT (Disco-CT) in Percutaneous Discectomy

M. LUTZE and H. M. MAYER [1]

Introduction

The improvement in radiological diagnosis of lumbar disc disease achieved by the development of spinal computerized tomography and by quantitative magnetic resonance imaging has increased the reliability of patient selection for percutaneous discectomy.

Although discography [8, 13] had originally gained wide recognition it largely lost its significance due to the development of contrast media for myelography and due to CT and MRI. Recently discography experienced a renaissance as a perioperative procedure associated with percutaneous treatment (chemonucleolysis, percutaneous discectomy) of lumbar disc disease [3, 7, 11, 14, 18, 21].

While some authors still emphasize its value in the differential diagnosis of lumbar syndromes, e.g. prior to fusion procedures [6, 9], others suggest that discography be relegated to the "hall of fame of bygone radiologic techniques" [1, 5, 16, 19, 20].

Occasional difficulties in the interpretation of spinal CT [16] led to the idea of obtaining axial images of lumbar discograms by performing postdiscographic CT scans [15]. These permit a more precise localization of annular defects as well as of protrusions and of disc fragments [4, 16, 24]. A number of prospective studies substantiate the value of postdiscographic CT images in demonstrating intra- and extraforaminal disc protrusions and in differentiating them from enlarged roots, ganglia, or tumors [2, 10, 12]. In addition, the axial imaging facilitates the recognition of artifacts caused by non-nuclear, annular or epidural injections [15].

A major contribution towards classification of the "discography CT" was made by the group of Mooney [17], which developed a new classification, the "Dallas Discogram Description", on the basis of five different parameters: "degeneration", "annular disruption", "pain response", "contrast volume", "miscellaneous information". These authors consider disco-CT to be a highly sensitive method which permits detection of even minimal alterations in disc morphology not visible in myelography, computerized tomography, routine discography, and even MRI.

Subsequent investigations of these authors show a close relationship between ruptures of the anulus and the reproduction of pain radiation during discography,

---

[1] Abteilung für Neurochirurgie, Klinikum Steglitz, Freie Universität, Berlin, Hindenburgdamm 30, 1000 Berlin 45, FRG

Percutaneous Lumbar Discectomy
Ed. by H. M. Mayer and M. Brock

but no significant correlation between discography, computed tomography, pain response and reduction of intervertebral disc height [22, 23].

We have been using disco-CT in order to achieve a more refined indication for percutaneous discectomy. In this paper we report on our initial experience with this method.

Material and Methods

Twenty-one discography CTs were performed in 20 patients (12 men and 8 women) in the time period extending from Jan. 6, 1988 to Oct. 15, 1988. The age ranged between 21 and 64 years (mean: 45 years in males and 49 years in females). The distribution of investigated levels was as follows: L 3/4 (n = 5), L 4/5 (n = 13), L 5/S 1 (n = 3).

Discography was performed with Solutrast 250 M® (Iopamidol; Fa. Byk Gulden, Konstanz, FRG), using the posterolateral approach described in detail elsewhere [3, 14].

Results

There was a medium- to high-grade of disc degeneration in 3 cases, a protrusion with partial rupture of the anulus fibrosus in 7 cases (4 lateral, 3 paramedian), a subligamentous deposit of contrast-medium in 4, and a "free" perforation in 7 (2 paramedian, 4 intraforaminal, 1 extraforaminal) (Fig. 1). All patients suffered from subacute or chronic sciatica and low back pain and had previously been submitted to myelography and/or computed tomography, but the radiological findings either did not agree with the symptoms or suggested a lateral prolapse.

The indication for disco-CT was established on the basis of the necessity to differentiate between protrusion (annulus intact!) and a prolapse (annulus ruptured). Moreover, disco-CT should help to delineate the border of the disc-herni-

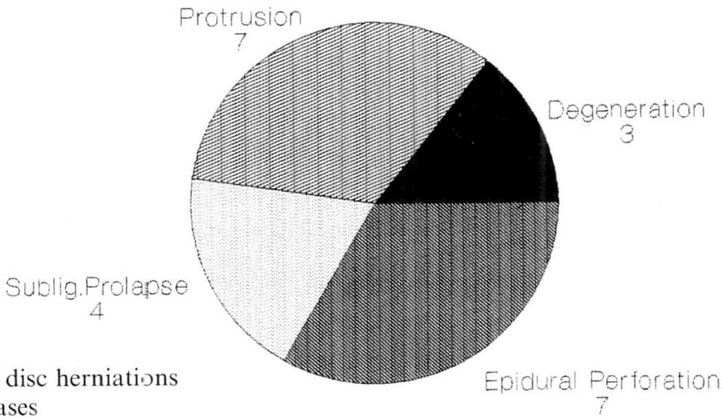

Fig. 1. Pathomorphology of disc herniations verified by disco-CT in 20 cases

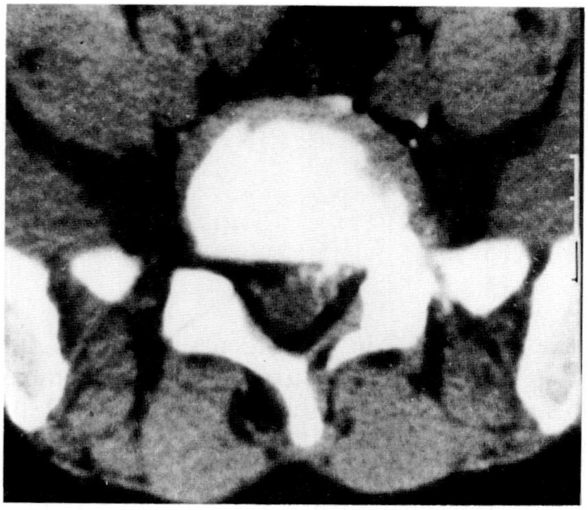

Fig. 2. Disco-CT demonstrating a perforated intraforaminal prolapse at L 4/5. The contrast medium leaks out of the disc space into the foramen and backwards into the epidural space

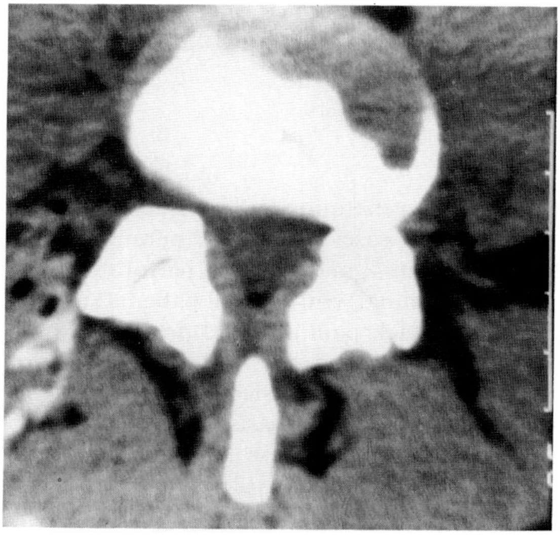

Fig. 3. Disco-CT showing an intraforaminal disc protrusion without leakage of the contrast medium beyond the annulus fibrosus

ation from the anatomical structures in the neighborhood (nerve-root, ganglion, epidural space). Twelve patients of our series were submitted to an "open" surgical procedure (interlaminar fenestration, hemilaminectomy) (Fig. 2) and 3 to percutaneous discectomy. Five patients continued to receive conservative treatment. The interval between disco-CT and operation was up to 24 hours. Preoperative diagnosis based on disco-CT was confirmed at surgery in all patients.

Among the 4 patients with lateral protrusions, one underwent percutaneous discectomy, one continued to receive conservative therapy (in view of the symptoms being regressive), one had a narrow spinal canal with spondylosis deformans, and one was not eligible for percutaneous discectomy because the level was L 5/S 1.

Of the three patients with paramedian protrusions, two women were submitted to percutaneous discectomy (Fig. 3) while in the third, disco-CT demonstrated a narrow lateral recess bilaterally.

The three patients submitted to percutaneous discectomy were nearly completely free of radicular symptoms following the procedure.

Discussion

These preliminary results do not as yet permit definitive statements on the value of disco-CT in predicting the results of percutaneous discectomy. A descriptive classification such as the "Dallas Discogram Description" seems to be of a more academic character and to have little practical value for pecutaneous discectomy. However, disco-CT is the most sensitive and reliable method to exclude a disc prolapse perforated or sequestrated beyond the dorsal longitudinal ligament, which is one of the main contraindications for percutaneous discectomy.

Discography surely has its place as a routine procedure prior to the performance of percutaneous discectomy, since it permits perioperative a/p and lateral demonstration of disc pathomorphology, measurement of the nuclear resistance and the possible triggering of a "memory pain" [14].

Postdiscographic CT scans have proven to be a valuable aid in the exact visualization of the degree of degeneration and the "rupture course" of the dorsal anulus fibrosus. The same is true for the differentiation between lateral, intra- and extraforaminal disc prolapse, which may be improved by CT reconstruction procedures. However, care should be taken to exclude artifacts [15] due to misleading contrast-medium injections outside the nucleus. This can be avoided by the exact positioning of the discography cannula in the geometric center of the intervertebral space.

References

1. Abdelwahab IF, Gould ES (1988) The role of discography after negative postmyelography CT scans. AJNR 9:187–190
2. Angtuaco EJC et al. (1984) Computed tomographic discography in the evaluation of extreme lateral disc herniation. Neurosurgery 14:350–352
3. Brock M, Mayer HM, Görge HH (1984) Die Chemonukleolyse mit Chymopapain. Deutsches Ärzteblatt 81:2965–2970
4. Edwards WC, Orme IT, Orr-Edwards G (1987) CT discography: Prognostic value in the selection of patients for chemonucleolysis. Spine 12/8:792–795
5. Gibson MJ et al. (1986) Magnetic resonance imaging and discography in the diagnosis of disc degeneration. J Bone Joint Surg 68-13:369–373
6. Grubb SA, Lipscomb HJ, Guilford WB (1987) The relative value of lumbar roentgenograms, metrizamide myelography, and discography in the assessment of patients with chronic low-back syndrome. Spine 12/3:282–286
7. Hijikata SA (1975) A method of percutaneous nuclear extraction. J X Toden Hospital 5:39
8. Holt EP (1968) The question of lumbar discography. J Bone Joint Surg 50-A:720–726

9. Hsu KI et al. (1988) Painful lumbar end-plate disruptions: A significant discographic finding. Spine 13/1:76–78
10. Jackson RP, Glah II (1987) Foraminal and extraforaminal lumbar disc herniation: Diagnosis and treatment. Spine 12/6:577–585
11. Kambin P, Gellmann H (1983) Percutaneous lateral discectomy of the lumbar spine. Clin Orth Rel Res 174:127–132
12. Kornberg M (1987) Computed tomography of the lumbar spine following discography. Spine 12/8:823–825
13. Lindblom K (1948) Diagnostic puncture of intervertebral disc in sciatica. Acta Orthop Scand 17:231–239
14. Mayer HM, Brock M (1988) Die perkutane Diskektomie. Dtsch Ärzteblatt 85:853–858
15. McCutcheon ME, Thompson III WC (1986) CT scanning of lumbar discography. Spine 11/3:257–259
16. Modic MT et al. (1988) Imaging of degenerative disc disease. Radiology 168:177–186
17. Sachs BL et al. (1987) Dallas discogram description. A new classification of CT/discography in low-back disorders. Spine 12/3:287–294
18. Schleberger R, Kolditz D, Krämer I (1985) Der Stellenwert der Diskographie bei lumbaler Bandscheibenlockerung. Orthop Praxis 4:296–299
19. Schneidermann G et al. (1987) Magnetic resonance imaging in the diagnosis of disc degeneration: Correlation with discography. Spine 12/3:276–281
20. Shapiro R (1986) Current status of lumbar discography. Radiology 159/3:815
21. Troisier O, Cypel D (1986) Discography: An element of decision. Surgery versus chemonucleolysis. Clin Orth Rel Res 206:70–78
22. Vanharanta H et al. (1987) The relationship of pain provocation to lumbar disc deterioriation as seen by CT/discography. Spine 12/3:295–298
23. Vanharanta H et al. (1988) A comparison of CT/discography, pain response and radiographic disc height. Spine 13/3:321–324
24. Videman T, Malmivaara A, Mooney V (1987) The value of the axial view in assessing discograms. Spine 12/3:299–304

Prospective Evaluation of Correlations Between Discomanometry and MR Imaging Data: Role in the Management of Disc Disease – Preliminary Results

L. CASTAGNERA [1], N. GRENIER [2], B. LAVIGNOLLE [1], J. M. CAILLE [2], and J. SENEGAS [1]

In the past, percutaneous nucleotomy (PN) indications did not seem to have been clearly defined and its success rate, commonly of 75%–80%, draws near to chemonucleolysis (CN) results published in the literature. However, in recent years, more accurate definition of CN indications has given rise to significantly improved CN results and a success rate of 95%, with respect to certain discographic data [3]. In the same way, a CN success rate of more than 98% can be obtained with respect to specific discomanometric data [2]. Discomanometry (DMM) is a physical investigation of the disc which consists of evaluation of its compliance status. Its diagnostic value has been demonstrated [1, 2], permitting recognition of leaking from "non-leaking" discs, and assessment and quantification of the degree of disc degeneration in terms of discal pressure level and volume of fluid tolerated by the disc. Its predictive value is based on significant correlation between its data and CN results [2]. It follows therefrom that, as for CN, DMM had to be performed before PN procedure. Consequently, PN results had to be assessed in accordance with the data of DMM.

Magnetic resonance imaging (MRI) has a diagnostic value. It can show longitudinal ligament integrity or disruption in disc herniation [5]; it can evaluate hydration status of the disc which has been reported to be related to its degenerative level [6, 8, 9].

The purpose of the present study is to correlate the DMM and MRI data and to correlate these with PN results in order to attempt to specify PN indications.

Methods

Between February 1 and July 1, 1988, thirty seven patients (M/F: 25/12), suffering from sciatic radiculopathy were scheduled to PN procedure with respect to clinical and CT scan criteria (non-migrated protruded or herniated discs).

MRI was performed preoperatively on 28/37 patients on a 0.5 tesla magnet (Magniscan 5000, General Electric CGR) with a surface coil for spine imaging. Two types of sequences were achieved: T1-weighted (TR = 500, TE = 26 ms) on sagittal and axial view and T2-weighted (TR = 2000, TE = 40 ms and 4 echos) on the sagittal only. The studied factors were: 1) Volume of the herniation (VH)

[1] Service de Chirurgie de la Colonne Vertébrale, [2] Service de Radiologie, Hôpital Pellegrin Tripode, 33076 Bordeaux Cedex, France

Percutaneous Lumbar Discectomy
Ed. by H. M. Mayer and M. Brock

assessed by measuring its 3 dimensions; 2) Percentage of disc height loss (% HL) compared to normal; 3) Percentage of signal intensity loss (% SIL) compared to normally hydrated discs. Signal intensity was measured by regions of interest (ROI) on the second echo (TE = 80 ms) of the long TR sequence. Each patient was his or her own reference at a normal disc level.

DMM was performed on a total of 53 discs in the 37 patients, in the operating room, just before PN procedure. Patients were placed in the lateral decubitus position. A (22 G) needle is introduced posterolaterally, under local anesthesia, into the center of the disc. Good positioning of the needle is controlled by lateral and anteroposterior X-rays. After correct localization, the needle is connected to a three-way stopcock. One way is connected, by means of a rigid polyethylene tube, to a kit used for this study (Société Galtier, Montpellier, France) and made of a transducer capable of handling more than 7500 mmHg related to a special paper recorder. The second way is connected to a syringe handled by the operator. The whole apparatus is filled with isotonic saline solution. The proper method consists of injecting 0.9% NaCl solution into the center of the disc in two phases: 0.5 first, then 1 ml 10 s later. The evolution of the intradiscal pressure induced is recorded during 60 s from the moment of the second injection. The studied factors were: 1) pressure level at 0 and 60 s (P 0; P 60); 2) pressure loss at zero and 60 s (% P 0; % P 60) with reference to pressure obtained in normal disc with the same method; 3) decrease of the measured area under the curve with reference to normal (% S); 4) discal volume (DV), i.e. the quantity of fluid injected into the disc that induced the patient's leg pain in a patient with a symptomatic disc. Then each disc could be classified according to the classification previously described [1, 2]. This can be summarized as follows: Group I consists of non-leaking (P 60 > 0) and symptomatic discs (DV +). It is subdivided into 4 types (A, B, C, D) by reference to P 60 (which significantly decreases from IA to ID) and DV values (which significantly increase from IA to ID, proportionately to P 60 decrease). The pressure curves show a low and regular curve slope. Group II also consists of non-leaking and symptomatic discs (P 60 > 0; DV +). However, they are characterized by irregular decrease of the discal pressure; the pressure curves reveal a high slope. Group III consists of non-leaking discs with low P 60 (205 ± 52 mmHg). These are not symptomatic discs (DV–) despite filling volume superior to 4 ml. Group IV consists of ruptured discs (P 60 = 0) characterized by an abrupt decrease of the discal pressure.

The PN procedure was achieved in the operating room, under local anesthesia, on patients in the lateral decubitus position, at the level determined in accordance with clinical, CT scan, DMM and MRI data. The PN technique was practically similar to the one used by Kambin [7]. Results were analyzed immediately and, at mid-term, according to Suezawa and Schreiber score [12].

Statistical Analysis

DMM and MRI data were expressed in terms of mean (X) ± SD and compared using a Student test. Correlation was established between MRI and DMM quantitative data, between MRI data and PN results, and between DMM data and PN results (Spearman correlation). PN results were analyzed after 2 months and compared according to DMM data by using the exact probability Fisher test. Statistical significance was defined as $p \leq 0.05$.

Results

Correlation Between DMM and MRI Data (Tables 1 and 2): Among 28 patients studied by both DMM and MRI methods, thirty six discs could be assessed: 24 at L4–L5, 12 at L5–S1. Means, extreme values and standard deviation for all DMM and MRI data are shown in Table 1. The comparative study reveals that DMM factors (% P0, % S) are comparable with % SIL given by MRI (p=NS). However, no correlation could be found between these (r=0.2 to 0.4; p=NS) (Table 2).

All DMM factors are strongly related to each other ($p<0.05$ to $p<0.0001$), while none of MRI factors are related (r=0.0 to 0.3; p=NS).

Correlation Between DMM and MRI Data and PN Results (Tables 3 and 4): PN procedure was performed on 37 patients and 37 discs were treated at one level (30 at L4–L5; 7 at L5–S1). Neither infection nor neurologic or vascular damage was noted.

The PN results are shown in Table 3 according to DMM classification. The correlation study is shown in Table 4 PN success (Table 3) decreases proportionately to P60 decrease and DV increase. The best results are obtained in types IA (Group I) and in Group II. Good results decrease from IA to IC; no type ID could be assessed. PN success is comparable in Groups I and II (p=NS); excellent and good results seem better in Group II, but no difference was found (p=NS). PN procedure gave one good result in Group III (totally degenerated discs). In Group IV, it gave a good result despite a ruptured disc proved on DMM, then on discography.

Table 1. Descriptive analysis of DMM and MRI data

DMM data	PO [mm Hg]	PO [%]	P60 [mm Hg]	P60 [%]	S [%]	DV [ml]
X̄ ±SD	1230.4 ±367.9	49.2 ±14.7	594.6 ±371.2	25.2 ±14.6	41.7 ±12.8	1.8 ±0.9
	(150→1800)	(6→72)	(100→1350)	(2→54)	(4.2→70)	(0.5→3.5)
MRI data	**VH [ml]**	**HL [%]**	**SIL [%]**			
X̄ ±SD	0.31 ±0.15	85.4 ±12.4	48.75 ±19.1			
	(0.11→0.64)	(55→100)	(20.4→94.8)			

Table 2. Correlations between DMM data and MRI data (r=coefficient of correlation; * $p<0.05$, ** $p<0.01$, *** $p<0.001$)

	PO (r)	% P60 (r)	% S (r)	DV (r)	VH (r)	% HL (r)	% SIL (r)
PO, % PO	0.49**	0.64***	0.87***	0.44*	0.3 (NS)	0.0 (NS)	0.2 (NS)
P60		0.85***	0.618***	0.44*	0.2 (NS)	0.0 (NS)	0.1 (NS)
% P60			0.639***	0.44*	0.2 (NS)	0.1 (NS)	0.1 (NS)
% S				0.42*	0.3 (NS)	0.0 (NS)	0.3 (NS)
DV					0.1 (NS)	0.1 (NS)	0.0 (NS)
VH						0.2 (NS)	0.1 (NS)
% HL							0 (NS)

Table 3. PN results on 37 patients according to DMM classification

	Exc	Good	Fair	Poor
Group I (n=22)	3	14	4	1
IA	1	1	–	–
IB	2	4	1	–
IC	–	9	3	–
ID	–	–	–	–
Group II (n=11)	–	10	–	1
Group III (n=3)	–	1	1	1
Group IV (n=1)	–	1	–	–

Table 4. Study of correlations (r) between DMM, MRI data and PN results

		PN results	
DMM datas	PO	r=0.6	p<0.0001
	P60	r=0.45	p<0.008
	% P60	r=0.53	p<0.001
	% S	r=0.537	p<0.001
	DV	r=0.48	p<0.005
MRI datas	VH	r=0.34	p=NS
	% HL	r=0.038	p=NS
	% SIL	r=0.1	p=NS

A strong correlation could be established between DMM factors (P0 or % P0, P60, % S, DV) and PN results, whether together ($r=0.6$, $p<0.001$) or individually ($0.05<p<0.0001$), as shown in Table 4.

Among the 28 patients who benefited from MRI, no correlation could be found between MRI factors and PN results (p=NS).

Discussion

PN clinical and imaging indications appear similar to those of CN, but do not seem to be clearly defined. The patient selection for PN procedures does not appear accurate enough, since the mean success rate draws near to 75–80%. The complementary investigations performed to date, do not seem reliable enough to permit a satisfactory selection and consequently do not increase PN success rate. The actual problem concerning indications of PN resembles that of CN some years ago: At that period, CN success rate was about 75%. Actually, it can be superior to 95% if some discographic data are acknowledged [3]; it is more than 98% for those patients whose discs were of high pressure and low DV ($P60>600$ mmHg; $DV\leq 2.5$ ml) according to DMM findings [2]. Thus, what was done to make CN indications more precise deserved to be studied with regard to PN indications. Therefore, we decided to evaluate the benefit of DMM and MRI regarding this last point. In our opinion, on considering selection for PN procedure, three questions had to be resolved:

1. Is the posterior longitudinal ligament (PLL) ruptured? 2. Does a herniated fragment communicate with the center of the disc? Indeed a non-ruptured PLL and the existence of a good communication between the disc and the fragment seem to be the two conditions necessary for the reinstatement of herniation into the cavity created by nucleotomy. 3. What is the degree of disc degeneration? We wanted to emphasize this problem because we think a preoperative evaluation of disc degeneration can contribute to standardization of PN indications, and probably to determination of PN results.

All the imaging or physical diagnostic methods need to be discussed in order to answer these three questions. Discography is able to show a disc herniation and to assess integrity or disruption of the PLL, but false negatives exist because iodine contrast medium cannot always diffuse to the herniation [4]. MRI can show rupture of the PLL on short TR/TE and long TR/short TE images on the sagittal view when correlated with surgical findings [5]. DMM can predict PLL disruption (group IV discs), and correlation had been previously established with discography [1]. In our series, correlation was achieved between MRI and DMM: When compared with DMM, MRI overestimated PLL disruption.

Discography alone, or combined with CT scan, can demonstrate the presence of a good communication between disc and herniation, but only in 52% of the cases [13]. Therefore, false absence of visualization of communication is a problem with this method. DMM cannot visualize this communication, but permits an assessment of the symptomatic character of a disc. The induced pain has a diagnostic [2, 11, 13] and prognostic [1, 2, 13] value, and suggests indirectly a communication between the disc and the hernia. The pain is always induced by using isotonic saline solution during DMM in the case of a symptomatic disc, while it may not be apparent in 45% of cases by using iodine contrast medium [13]. This can be explained by the high viscosity and thus the lesser capacity of diffusion of contrast in comparison to saline solution. The communication of the herniated fragment with the center of the disc is impossible to recognize with MRI because the nucleus pulposus can never be separated from the inner annulus fibers, whatever sequence one uses [9]. Both have the same signal intensity, and the only separation one can observe is between inner fibers and outer fibers of the annulus.

MRI is the only imaging technique allowing a quantification of degeneration in terms of hydration level according to the signal intensity observed on long TR/TE images [8, 9]. DMM is a non-imaging technique quantifying the degree of disc degeneration in terms of pressure level and discal tolerance volume [1]. Therefore, we wanted to know if disc degeneration could be equally quantified by MRI and DMM, to decide if that could help in patient selection for PN procedure and evaluation of PN results.

The absence of correlation between the pressure level (measured during DMM) and hydration level (measured by the signal intensity loss on T2 weighted images) was surprising but somewhat understandable. These results mean that pressure and hydration are not correlated factors, which is confirmed by MRI images obtained after PN: In the three cases we imaged 48 h after PN, no change of signal intensity could be identified while intradiscal pressure is known to decrease after PN [10]. The lack of correlation between MRI and PN results compared to the significant correlation between PN and DMM data means that results of percutaneous decompression are indeed related to the intradiscal pressure, but not to the hydration level of the disc. Therefore, we think that the degree of disc degeneration for PN patient selection must be assessed in terms of pressure level and not in terms of hydration of the disc for the effectiveness of this therapeutic method. Moreover, it seems logical to suppose that since the PN principle consists of discal decompression, its results will be all the better when that pressure is raised. That is what appears in this preliminary study: In high pressure discs (type IA, Group I), PN results were good in all cases and the number of good results decreases in parallel to the diminution of pressure, as shown by significant correlation between these factors.

In conclusion, the level of disc degeneration shown by MRI is poorly correlated with that measured by DMM. However, correlation has to be pursued on a larger population with external intensity standard for MRI signal intensity measurement in order to use the same "gold standard" for each patient.

To date, DMM is the only method which has proved to be correlated with PN results. Its predictive value enables it to be considered as a reliable method to select PN indications. DMM can be considered as a reference method. On a statistical point of view, its quantitative and measurable data permit the identification of each disc and each group of discs, and comparison of results of percutaneous techniques (CN, PN, automated percutaneous lumbar discectomy).

References

1. Castagnera L, LaVignolle B, Claverie JP, Vital JM, Baulny D, Senegas J (1987) Test de tolérance discale et discomanométrie. Intérêt diagnostique et pronostique avant chimionucléolyse. Acta Orthop Belg 53:184–194
2. Castagnera L, LaVignolle B, Vital JM, Grenier F, Baulny D, Senegas J (1987) Etude fonctionnelle du disque pathologique par la discomanométrie. Intérêt diagnostique et pronostique avant nucléolyse. Revue du Rhumatisme 55(5): 381–388
3. Edwards W, Orme T, Orr-Edwards B (1987) CT discography: Prognostic value in the selection of patients for chemonucleolysis. Spine 12:792–795
4. Frot B, Folinais D, Bourgeois P, Roger B (1988) Interêt de la discoscanographie lombaire dans les chymonucléolyses. Communication au Symposium sur l'approche percutanée des disques lombaires, Blois 4–5 mars 1988, Abstract p 54–58
5. Grenier N, Greselle JF, Vital JM et al. (1988) MR of lumbar longitudinal ligament. Normal anatomy and diagnosis of disruption in disc disease. Radiology (In press)
6. Jenkins JPR, Hickey DS, Zhu XP, Machin BA, Isherwood I (1985) MR imaging of the intervertebral disc: A quantitative study. Br J Radiol 58:705–709
7. Kambin P, Brager MD (1987) Percutaneous posterolateral discectomy. Clin Orth Rel Research 223:145–153
8. Modic MT, Pavlicek W, Weinstein MA et al. (1984) Magnetic resonance imaging of intervertebral disc. Clinical and pulse sequence considerations. Radiology 152:103–111
9. Modic MT, Masaryk TJ, Ross JS, Carter JR (1988) Imaging of degenerative disk disease. Radiology 168:177–186
10. Sakamoto T, Tajima K (1988) La difference des pressions intradiscales avant et après la nucléotomie percutanée. Communication au Symposium sur l'approche percutanée des disques lombaires, Blois 4–5 mars 1988, Abstract p 69–70
11. Shepperd J (1988) Discectomie percutanée. Communication au Symposium sur l'approche percutanée des disques lombaires, Blois, France, 4–5 mars, Abstract p 66–67
12. Suezawa Y, Schreiber A (1987) Komplexe Indikationen in der Chirurgie des Spinalkanals. Z Ortho 125:308–319
13. Troisier O, Cypel D (1987) Chirurgie ou nucléolyse? La discographie est-elle un facteur de décision? Acta Orthop Belg 53:195–203

Results of Magnetic Resonance Imaging (MRI) Investigation Before and After Automated Percutaneous Lumbar Discectomy (APLD) – Comparison of MRI Findings and Clinical Health Status

C. JANTEA [1], J. ASSHEUER [2], K. SCHÖPPE [1], and K.P. SCHULITZ [1]

Degenerative changes of the lumbar disc are part of the general process of aging [16].

An imbalance of mechanical stress and stress tolerance frequently results in a dorsal disc herniation which can be classified according to the shape of the discogram [1]. We took this staging one step further at our hospital by doing a distension test at the time of injection of dye into the disc, followed by a CAT-scan of the injected disc (disco-CT) [25]. When clinical symptoms and radiological findings (disco-CT, MRI) suggested a contained disc, we felt that percutaneous nucleotomy (APLD) was indicated. This procedure, which was introduced by Onik and Maroon in 1985 [22], is essentially a very gentle kind of surgery for a disease which was described by Mixter and Barr in 1934. The latter authors suggested open discectomy as the treatment of choice [20]. Magnetic resonance imaging (MRI) soon established itself as a routine method of diagnosing lumbar spinal disease [26]. In contrast to more conventional techniques (CAT scan, discography, myelography) MRI offers the advantage of pictures in a sagittal, coronal and transverse plane without potentially hazardous radiation. In addition, it does not only show morphological changes but also, to a certain extent, functional changes by measuring the differences in resonance of protons in the relaxation phase [2, 23].

The aim of our study was to find answers to the following questions:

- Which morphological changes can be found when comparing MRI of discs before and after APLD?
- Does the degree of degeneration of the disc before and after APLD correlate with the clinical symptoms?

Material and Methods

A. Magnetic resonance imaging (MRI). MRI is based upon the effects of resonance of protons. These activated protons are given a certain direction by a strong external magnetic field. Then they are pushed into another direction by a short

[1] Orthopädische Universitätsklinik, Moorenstr. 5, 4000 Düsseldorf 1, FRG
[2] Institut für Radiologie und Kernspintomographie, Genovevastr. 24, 5000 Köln, FRG

Percutaneous Lumbar Discectomy
Ed. by H.M. Mayer and M. Brock

high frequency impulse. Two factors contribute towards a return to the old direction:

- the thermic link of the nuclei to their surroundings, characterized by T 1
- the mutual influences of the nuclei, characterized by T 2.

The initial signal depends on the number of activated protons. The rate of decrease depends on their relaxation times. The main difference between MRI and other visualizing techniques is the fact that resonance signals give some information about certain biological functions [27]. Because the content of free water in the disc is higher than in the bone marrow, the T 2 relaxation time is longer in the disc. Thus T 2-weighted sequences are very appropriate to differentiate these two components. Since we did not anticipate this fact initially, we mainly used T 1-weighted ($T1 = 400-800$ ms, $T2 = 20-50$ ms) and moderately T 2-weighted sequences ($T1 = 1600-2000$ ms, $T2 = 60-100$ ms) in our study. Our MRI investigations were done on a 0.15-tesla and later on a 1.00-tesla scanner by Picker.

In order to directly compare our findings in a patient before and after APLD, we had to standardize our imaging technique. We finally succeeded in achieving optimal scans parallel to the endplates of all segments including L 4/5 and L 5/S 1. These scans were reproducible (Fig. 1). In addition to sagittal cuts, we did cuts in coronal and frontal planes as well. We used the same standardized sequences pre- and postoperatively.

In order to assess the lumbar disc degeneration, we developed a numeric score which considered both morphological criteria and tissue-related resonance parameters (Table 1).

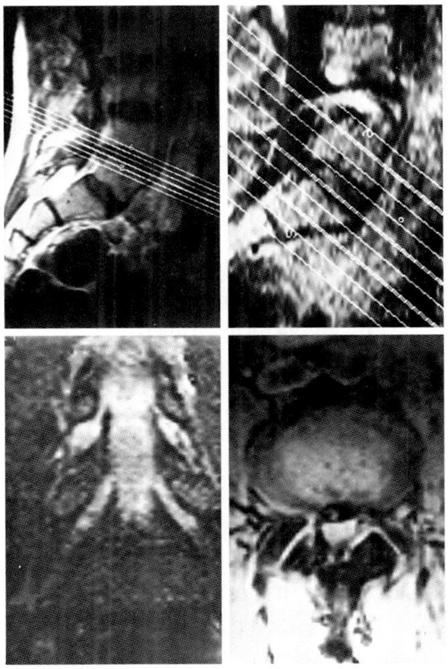

Fig. 1. Magnetic resonance imaging of lumbar spine. *Top:* standard sequence for intervertebral disc tissue ($T1 = 500$ ms, $T2 = 10$ ms). *Bottom:* T 2-weighted setting to show the dural sac and the branching spinal nerves in the coronal plane

Table 1. MRI disc degeneration score for lumbar discs. By adding up the individual points one obtains a disc degeneration score for each lumbar disc. The first two parameters are drawn from the standard sequences for lumbar discs, the last two criteria are derived from T2-weighted pictures

Type of Disc Extrusion	Density of Water
0 = physiologic status	0 = physiologic status
1 = symmetric protrusion	1 = slight reduction
2 = prolapse	2 = severe reduction
3 = free fragment	
Lumbar Disc-Height Ratio	Vertebral Body Reaction
0 = physiologic status	0 = physiologic status
1 = slight reduction	1 = slight reduction
2 = severe reduction	2 = severe reduction

Table 2. MOPO scales: measurement of patient outcome (after Jäckel). Eight scales (61 items) reflect the patient's state of health

Mobility	Pain
Physical activity	Depression
Household activity	Anxiety
Social activity	
Activities of daily living	

This score took four criteria into consideration:

- The type of disc extrusion;
- the height of the disc, adapted from Wackenheim's "theory of block vertebrae";
- the water content of the disc. The affected disc was compared to the healthy disc one level above;
- reactive changes of the vertebral body and the endplates.

Minor changes affecting up to one third of total vertebral height were given one point, major changes were given two points.

This resulted in a normal disc having no points at all. A score between 1 and 4 points marked moderate degeneration.

In each patient, MRI was performed before and after surgery.

B. Mopo scales. In order to monitor the health status of the patient before and after APLD, we used standardized MOPO scales. These MOPO scales of the lumbar spine according to Jäckel are basically modified AIMS scales (arthritis impact measurement scales) of Boston University (USA) [10, 11]. There are 8 scales with 61 items and in the end a total score is figured out for each individual scale. In addition, there is a total score which considers all scales (Table 2). The first five scales describe mobility parameters. This score is such that a high number of points implies a good function. In the last three scales (pain, depres-

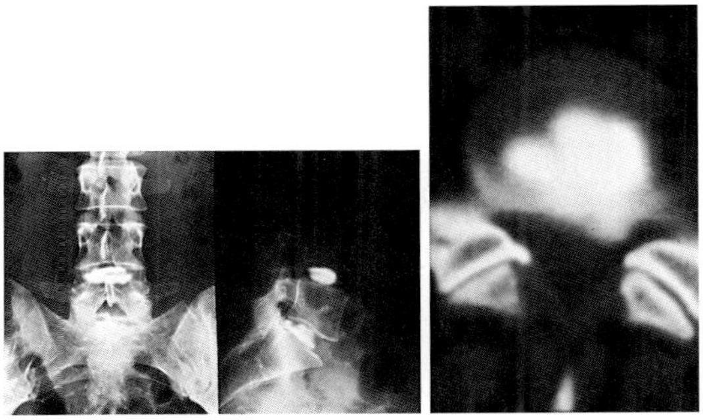

Fig. 2. Lumbar disc degeneration: contained disc with prolapse on the L 5/S 1 level, left-sided. Neither in the discogram nor in the CT scan thereafter (disco-CT) is a leak of contrast visualized. The 29-year-old female patient showed full remission of monoradicular symptoms after APLD on the L 5/S 1 level

sion, and anxiety), high scores are pathological. For this reason we multipied the number of points of the last three scales by −1 when we figured out the score of all scales. We used these scales because we felt that classical parameters such as Schober's sign, Patrick's sign and straight leg raising sign have no significance in the patients' daily lives. Pain and considerable impairment due to loss of function are the factors that influence our patients' lives.

MOPO scales were recorded pre- and postoperatively.

Patients

As pointed out before, only those patients were considered appropriate for APLD who had a positive distension test at the time of discography, i.e. the patient had true sciatic pain when the dye was forcefully injected. In addition, both discography and disco-CT had to show a contained disc. This means that no leak of dye into the peridural space was allowed (Fig. 2). In the end we had 40 patients (14 females, 26 males) aged 22 to 78 years (mean 39.4 years) with 41 nucleotomies between March and June 1988. These herniated discs were localized in the segments L 3/4 (n = 1), L 4/5 (n = 19) and L 5/S 1 (n = 21). 11 patients required further surgery after APLD because of persisting symptoms. Our follow-up was between 2 and 6 months (mean 2.8 months).

Results

MRI

In Tables 3 and 4 we summarize the MRI findings before and after surgery in both groups of patients. There was no statistically significant difference between patients as far as disc extrusion was concerned. In those patients who had only APLD we found a symmetrical protrusion in 10 cases and a true herniation in 19

Table 3. Results of MRI examination as reflected by the MRI score (for details see text) of the operated lumbar discs before and after APLD in 29 patients

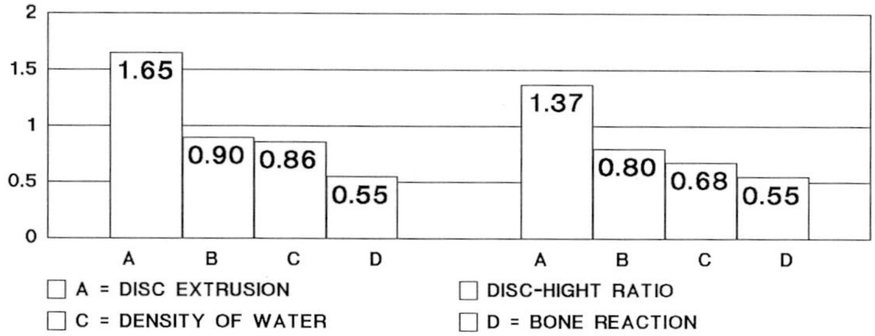

Table 4. Results of MRI examination as reflected by the MRI score of the operated lumbar discs before and after APLD plus open discectomy in 11 patients

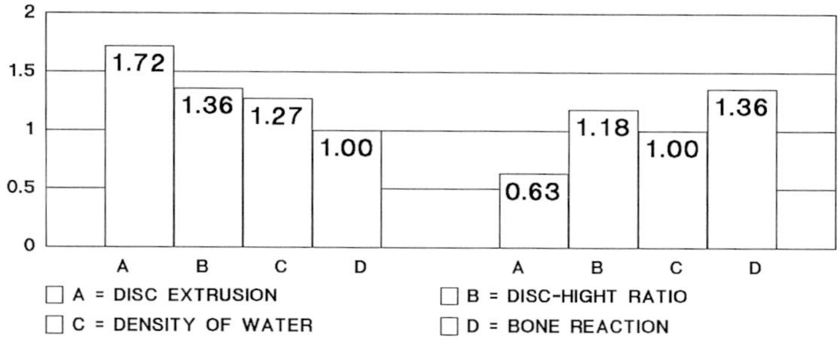

cases preoperatively. In those patients who had open surgery after APLD, we found 3 protrusions and 8 true herniations preoperatively.

When analyzing the postoperative MRI-pictures of the APLD group, we found slightly different relationships. In 18 patients we saw a symmetrical protrusion, and in 11 patients there was no change whatsoever. In those patients who had open surgery after APLD, we were unable to demonstrate a true herniation. In 7 cases, however, we found a symmetrical protrusion.

As far as our second morphological criterion was concerned, i.e. the height of the disc, we found the following results: before surgery in the APLD group there was 16 cases of slight, and 5 cases with severe loss of height. Postoperatively there were 13 cases with slight and 5 cases with severe loss of height. The summation score was preoperatively 0.90, postoperatively 0.80.

The average score in the second group of patients was 1.26 and after both APLD and open surgery it was 1.18. Preoperatively there was a slight loss of height in 3 patients, and a severe loss of height in 6 patients. Postoperatively, we found a slight loss of height in 3 patients and a severe loss in 5 patients.

As far as our third criterion, water content of the disc, was concerned, we found the following results: In our APLD group there were no pathological findings preoperatively in 12 patients, 9 patients had a slight reduction in water content, and 8 a severe one.

Their preoperative score was 0.86, and the postoperative score was 0.68. Postoperatively, 5 patients had a severe and 10 patient a slight reduction of the intradiscal water content. When analyzing the bony reaction, we found that in our APLD group (N=29) about one third of the cases (n=11) showed some bony reaction, 6 had a mild and 5 had severe changes which involved more than the marginal one third of the vertebral body. After APLD, 10 patients had mild and 3 patients had severe changes of their vertebral bony signals. Their summation score for this parameter did not change postoperatively at all. In our second group of patients (n=11), we found the following results: preoperatively there was a bony reaction in about two thirds of the cases (n=8), 5 were mild, and 3 were severe. After both APLD and open surgery we found positive reactions in ten patients: 5 were mild and 5 were severe. This explains why their score changes from 1.00 preoperatively to a worse 1.36 postoperatively.

MOPO-Scales

Tables 5 and 6 show the preoperative and postoperative score for each scale. Both groups had essentially the same initial mobility and activity scores. The score for mobility, for example, did not differ significantly from the group of patients who had only APLD, with a score of 4.72, and the group of patients who required open surgery thereafter. – Their score was 5.08. Interestingly enough, there was no change of the activity scales in either group of patients before and after surgery, nor were there significant changes in the scales pain, depression, and anxiety. This results in a preoperative summation score of 4.20 for the APLD group, and 4.28 for the APLD plus open surgery group.

Table 5. MOPO scales with demonstrating the patient's state of health before and after APLD. Third column shows scores of healthy volunteers (n=45)

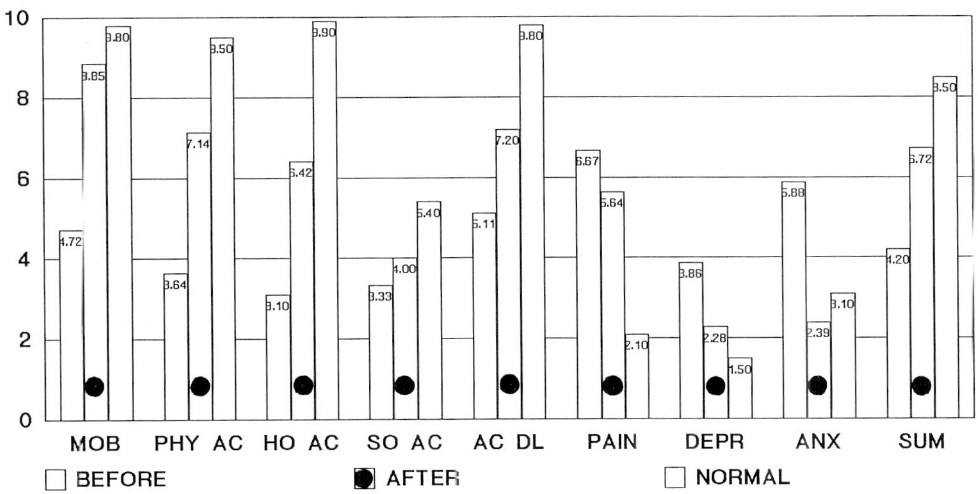

Table 6. MOPO scales: state of health of the 11 patients who required open surgery after APLD. First column: preoperative state; second column: state of health after both procedures; third column: state of health of asymptomatic volunteers

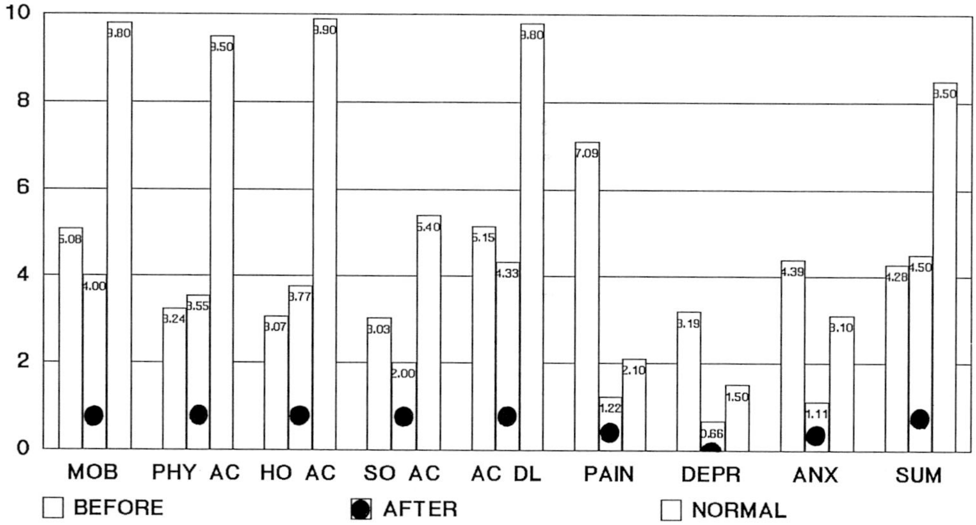

In the APLD group, there was a marked improvement of the score for activity (scale 1 to 5) postoperatively. Their average score ran at a 75% level of normal. As far as pain was concerned, their scores went from 6.67 to 5.64. This group of patients also showed the most significant reduction in depression (from 3.86 to 2.28) and anxiety (from 5.88 to 2.39). Their summation score rose from 4.2 preoperatively to 6.7 postoperatively. Our second group of patients (n = 11) did not show any significant changes in their mobility scale (scale 1–5). Much more interesting were the results of their scales 6–8. After both APLD and open surgery, their score went from 7.08 preoperatively to 1.22 postoperatively. Similarly, their scores for depression and anxiety decreased from 3.19 to 0.86 and 4.38 to 1.11, respectively. Their summation score, however, did not change significantly; it increased from 4.28 to 4.50.

Discussion

Studies of lumbar spinal degeneration have only a short tradition, historically. In 1932 Schmorl reported about 10000 dissections which he had performed personally [12, 15]. While the older publications concentrated on the bony morphology, more recent scientific papers developed a more sophisticated model of spinal degeneration by taking into consideration not only the actual bony changes, but also the causes and the consequences of those changes [5, 16]. It seems to become more and more clear that the etiology of acute sciatic pain, particularly in the older patient, is a very complex phenomenon in which not only visceral but also uni- or polymetamer reactions play a role [17].

Mechanical irritation of the root by herniated disc marterial with the classical radicular symptoms is, however, not trivial, as could be shown by Mixter and Barr [20].

Apart from a clinical neurological and orthopedic examination, diagnostic lumbar injection techniques (facet joint infiltrations, nerve blocks) have established themselves an appropriate method to reach a diagnosis [4, 7, 16].

The dynamic discography with subsequent computerized tomography helped us to make the diagnosis of a contained disc in the presence of sciatic pain (Fig. 2).

It were only those patients who were treated with APLD. We were unable to find any references which correlated MRI findings before and after percutaneous discectomy with a clinical score. Our postoperative findings demonstrated that in some cases, such as the one in Fig. 3, the disc does in fact decrease in size dorsally after surgery. We think that this phenomenon is due to an immediate gliding effect of posterior elements of the disc anteriorly after the operation, which then becomes permanent once scar tissue has formed [14].

This statement is supported by our own experiments in which we tried to remove dorsal subligamental parts of the disc through a typical posterolateral approach with standard instruments according to Hijikata (rigid tube) [9, 13] and with instruments designed by Onik and Maroon (flexible tube) [19, 22]. We were unable to reach the dorsal disc areas with either.

In cases like the one in Fig. 4 the shape of this herniation did not change macroscopically. However, the patient was pain-free immediately after the proce-

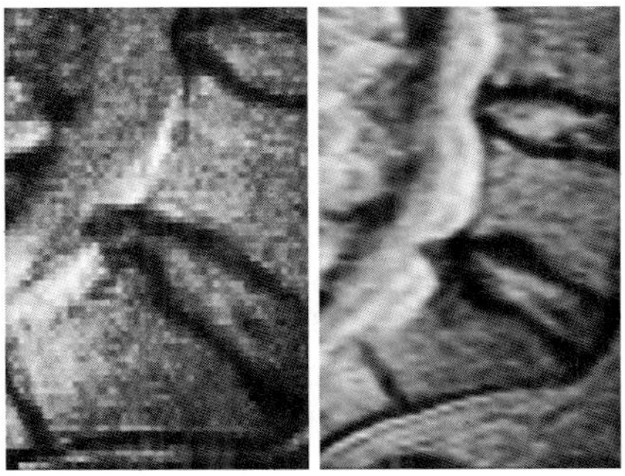

Fig. 3. Lumbar disc degeneration with median prolapse on the L 5/S 1 level in a 43-year-old female patient. *Left:* preoperative situation on MRI scan. *Right:* MRI control 14 days after APLD on the L 5/S 1 level. Note a slight reduction of prolapse size in the dorsal median area

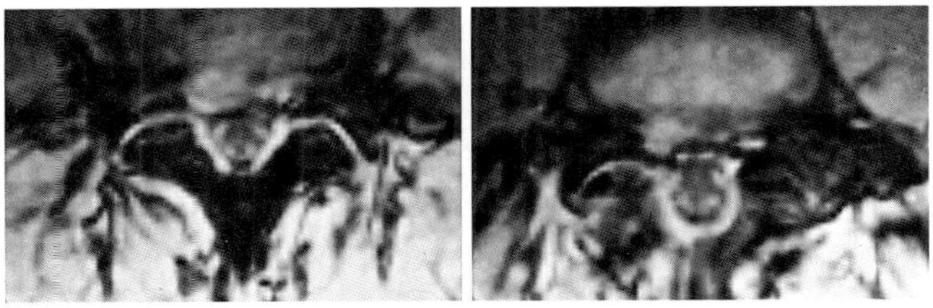

Fig. 4. Lumbar disc degeneration with lateral extrusion, L 4/5, left-sided, in a 27-year-old male patient. *Left:* preoperative status in MRI. *Right:* MRI control 11 days after APLD; there is no significant change of extrusion form, although this patient was free of symptoms after operation

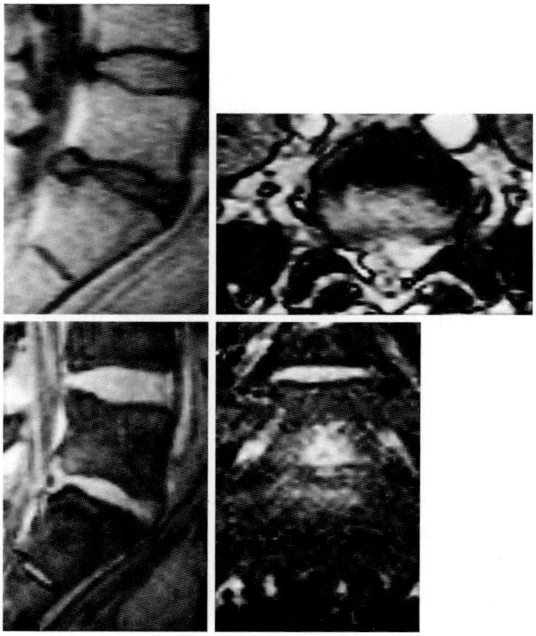

Fig. 5. Lumbar disc degeneration with median and left-sided prolapse on the L 5/S 1 level. *Top:* preoperative situation on MRI. *Bottom:* MRI control 81 days after APLD and open discectomy; prolapse configuration has disappeared. In the coronal tomogram, bone reaction (grade 2) of the basal half of the L 5 vertebral body and slight bone reaction (grade 1) of the dorsal area of S 1

dure. We think that this phenomenon is due to the fact that morphological changes of less than 1 mm cannot be demonstrated with the present day technique.

On the other hand, this surgical technique causes a denervation of the disc by destroying the intradiscal ends of the sinuvertebral nerves [3, 21, 24]. This latter phenomenon is certainly at least partially responsible for the decrease of lumbar muscle spasm and increasing mobility postoperatively. This increase in mobility could be objectively demonstrated both by manual examination according to Lewit, and radiologically [6, 18]. It is quite obvious that after open discectomy the herniation of the disc can not be demonstrated any more, as can be seen in Fig. 5. But even after open surgery, there were still minor protrusions which prevented the MRI score from going down from 1.7 preoperatively to 0.00. Instead, it went down to 0.63. Our second criterion of MRI analysis – disc height ratio – did not show any significant changes. Of course, one has to keep in mind that long-term results may differ like they do after chemical nucleolysis.

Our parameter "density of water" indicated a somewhat higher degree of dehydration of the disc in those patients who required open surgery (1.27 vs. 0.86), than in those who were treated with APLD alone.

The parameter "bony reaction" was very high in those 11 patients who required further surgery (1.00 vs. 0.55).

Figure 5 demonstrates a case in which preoperatively there was no bony reaction. Postoperatively, in contrast, in the moderately T 2-weighted sequences there were marked bony reactions in the upper endplate of S 1 as well as the dorsal part of the body of L 5. These changes are iatrogenic and due to intraoperative

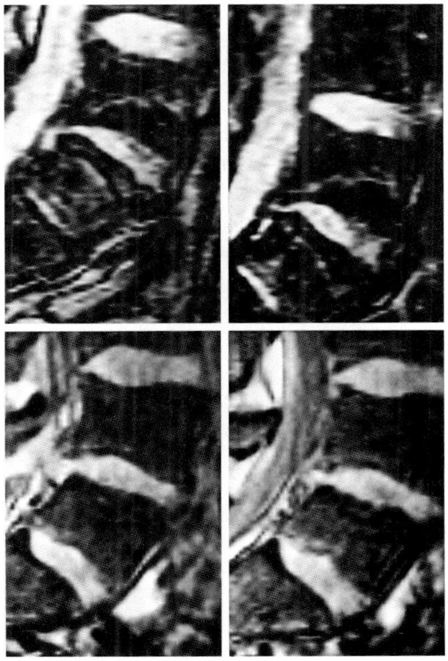

Fig. 6. Lumbar disc degeneration with median prolapse on the L 5/S 1 level and clinically asymptomatic protrusion on the L 4/5 level. *Top:* preoperative status in MRI. Please note the bone reaction (grade 2) of the bottom of the L 5 vertebra in the middle and anterior region. Slight reaction of S 1 vertebra (grade 1) in the marginal area of the endplate. *Bottom:* MRI control in the same 41-year-old female patient 220 days after APLD on the L 5/S 1 level. Note lack of bone reaction of the vertebral bodies

trauma. Clinically, this patient was completely pain-free at the time of his postoperative MRI.

A rather different finding can be seen on Fig. 6. In this case, it was a second-degree bony reaction in the neighboring endplates of L 5 and S 1. After APLD, these changes disappeared almost completely! In order to explain this phenomenon, we did transpedicular biopsies and found that histologically one can see fatty degenerative changes within the lymphocytic margin [26]. We thus assume that, after APLD, bony degenerative changes can regress. In our study, however, we could not demonstrate marked differences of this score parameter pre- and postoperatively, except for a few individual cases. This may be explained by our short-term follow-up.

It has been our intention to work out MRI criteria and clinical criteria which can predict the postoperative outcome of patients with discogenic disease. The standard MRI sequences are insufficient to allow these predictions. We are in the process of developing new sequences which will differentiate between fat and water more reliably.

The MOPO scales did not reveal any significant differences in either group of patients as far as physical health (scales 1–5) and psychological conditions were concerned (scale 6–8). Unlike other authors, we cannot confirm that poor results are due to psychological aspects of patients' personalities [8].

There was no significant correlation in our group of patients (n = 40) between MRI score and MOPO score. There was a tendency that those patients who required further surgery had a higher degree of disc degeneration preoperatively (MRI score 1.33), when compared to the APLD group alone (MRI score 0.99)

Table 7. MRI degeneration score of the operated segments before and after APLD in 29 patients and in 11 patients after APLD plus discectomy. (*Left:* preoperative status; *right:* post-operative status.) A = APLD; B = APLD and open discectomy

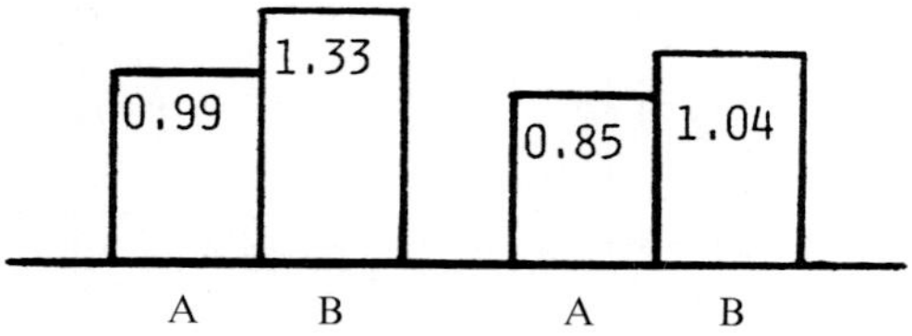

Table 8. Summation score of the state of health as measured by the MOPO scales. **a** = 29 patients who had APLD; **b** = 11 patients who had APLD plus discectomy; **c** = 45 healthy volunteers

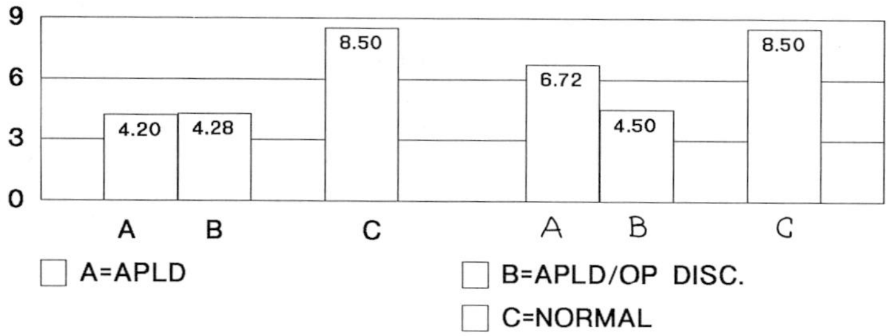

(Table 7). We were thus unable to predict the short-term postoperative outcome on the basis of classical criteria (such as neurological-orthopaedic examination), MRI or MOPO scales (Table 8).

The MOPO scales and our MRI score are useful instruments to describe and monitor spinal degenerative disease in a standardized way, helping to render comparable the results of both horizontal and longitudinal studies when lumbar disc surgery is performed by different investigators.

References

1. Adams MA, Dolan P, Hutton WC (1986) The stages of disc degeneration as revealed by discograms. JBJS 68(B): 34–41
2. Assheuer J, Lenz G, Lenz W, Gottschlich KW (1986) New aspects of degenerative intervertebral disc disease – the appearence in MR partial saturation and short time inversion recovery sequences. Nuc Compact 17: 4–8
3. Bogduk N, Windsor M, Inglis A (1988) The innervation of the cervical intervertebral discs. Spine 13(1): 2–8
4. Dooley JF, McBroom RJ, Taguchi T, Macnab I (1988) Nerve root infiltration in the diagnosis of radicular pain. Spine 13(1): 79–83
5. Edelson JG, Nathan H (1988) Stages in the natural history of the vertebral end-plates. Spine 13(1): 21–26

6. Gutmann G (1970) Klinisch-röntgenologische Untersuchung zur Statik der Wirbelsäule. In: Wolff HD (ed) Manuelle Medizin und ihre wissenschaftlichen Grundlagen. Verlag f. physik. Med., Heidelberg
7. Helbig T, Lee CK (1988) The lumbar facet syndrome. Spine 13(1): 61–78
8. Herron L, Tuner J, Weiner P (1988) Does the Minnesota Multiphasic Personality Inventory MMPI predict chemonucleolysis outcome? Spine 13(1): 84–88
9. Hijikata SA (1975) A method of percutaneous nuclear extraction. J Toden Hospital 5: 39
10. Jäckel W, Cziske R, Schohat T, Jacobi E (1986) Assessing health status after impatient rehabilitation in rheumatoid arthritis. Int Rehabil Med Eulars Publishers 8(2): 54–59
11. Jäckel W, Cziske R, Andres C, Jacobi E (1987) Messung der körperlichen Beeinträchtigung und der psychosozialen Konsequenzen bei chronischen Kreuzschmerzen. Z f Rheumatol 46: 25–33
12. Junghans H (1968) Die gesunde und die kranke Wirbelsäule in Röntgenbild und Klinik, 5 Aufl. Thieme, Stuttgart
13. Kambin P, Gellmann H (1983) Percutaneous lateral discectomy of lumbar spine. Clin Orth Rel Res 174: 127–132
14. Knapp K (1981) Die Wunde. Thieme, Stuttgart
15. Köhler A, Zimmer EA (1967) Grenzen des Normalen und Anfänge des Pathologischen im Röntgenbild des Skeletts, 11. Aufl. Thieme, Stuttgart New York
16. Krämer J (1986) Bandscheibenbedingte Erkrankungen, 2. Aufl. Thieme, Stuttgart
17. Kunert W (1975) Wirbelsäule und Innere Medizin, 2. Aufl. Enke, Stuttgart
18. Lewitt K (1988) Manuelle Medizin. Urban & Schwarzenberg, München
19. Maroon JC, Onik G (1987) Percutaneous automated discectomy; a new method for lumbar disc removal. J Neurosurg 66: 143–146
20. Mixter WJ, Barr JS (1934) Rupture of intervertebral disc with involvement of spinal canal. New Engl J Med 211: 210
21. Mulligan, cited by Kunert W (1975) Wirbelsäule und Innere Medizin, 2. Aufl. Enke, Stuttgart
22. Onik G, Helms CA, Linsberg L, Hoaglund ET, Morris J (1985) Percutaneous lumbar discectomy using a new aspiration probe. AJNR 6: 290–293
23. Ramm B, Semmler W, Laniaco M (1986) Einführung in die MR-Tomographie, Grundlagen und klinische Anwendung. Enke, Stuttgart
24. Rickenbacher J, Landolt AM, Theiler K (1982) Rücken. Springer, Berlin Heidelberg New York (Lanz T von, Wachsmuth W: Praktische Anatomie, Bd 2/7)
25. Schöppe K, Roggenland G, Schulitz KP (1988) The APLD method as a surgical treatment of lumbar disc herniation. Lecture on the Intern. Symposium on percutaneous lumbar discectomy in Berlin, August 12th, 1988
26. Schulitz KP, Assheuer J (1988) Die Bedeutung der Kernspin-Resonanztomographie für die Diagnose degenerativer Lendenwirbelsäulenerkrankungen. Z Orthop 126: 334–344
27. Steiner G, Fiegler W (1985) Kernspintomographie. Ecomed, Landsberg
28. Wackenheim A (1983) Röntgendiagnostik der Wirbel des Erwachsenen. Springer, Berlin Heidelberg New York

Percutaneous Lumbar Discectomy (PLD) – Technique and Results

Percutaneous Lumbar Discectomy – Indication, Technique and Results

P. KAMBIN [1]

The struggle to find an appropriate treatment for low back pain has been going on for centuries. Laminectomy, as a surgical means for the treatment of a herniated nucleus pulposus, became an acceptable procedure following Mixter and Barr's well-documented publication in the *New England Journal of Medicine* in 1934 [13].

Laminectomy remains the cornerstone for treatment of sequestrated discs and spinal stenosis. Certain undesirable complications associated with the laminectomy procedure have led investigators to search for an alternative method for surgical treatment of symptom-producing protruded intervertebral discs.

In 1951, Hult [1] described the anterior retroperitoneal approach for the evacuation and decompression of herniated lumbar discs. This approach is still being practiced in Japan. The concept of reduction of the volume of the nucleus by injection of chymopapain for the treatment of protruded lumbar discs was introduced by Lyman Smith in 1963 [15]. Since then, this procedure has been successfully utilized for the treatment of low back and sciatic pain. However, due to the inability of enzymes to digest the collagenized herniated nuclear fragments [16] and the reported complications, this procedure is losing its popularity, particularly in the United States.

Percutaneous lumbar discectomy offers an alternative method of treatment for lumbar radiculopathy due to a herniated disc [7–9]. Although the central evacuation and volume reduction, as well as large annular fenestration, plays an important role in the relief of pain following percutaneous lumbar discectomy, at this stage of the game we feel that the challenge of percutaneous lumbar discectomy lies in the capability of reaching posteriorly and evacuating the offending fragments [5].

The pathological examination of normal and protruded discs in fresh cadavers [3, 11] demonstrated that in the course of the degenerative process, the collagenized nuclear fragments may begin to migrate and often are trapped between the torn and entrapped annular fibers.

In skilled hands, the fear of causing neural injury in the course of this operative procedure seems to be unfounded. Although greater care should be exercised when attempting the L5–S1 disc extraction, one should have no difficulty in performing percutaneous discectomy at this level in most instances.

[1] The Graduate Hospital, Disc Treatment and Research Center, University of Pennsylvania, School of Medicine, Philadelphia, PA 19104, USA

Percutaneous Lumbar Discectomy
Ed. by H. M. Mayer and M. Brock

Indications

When surgical management becomes necessary, the physician has the responsibility to educate his or her patient about the various surgical modalities which are available, namely lumbar laminectomy, microlumbar discectomy, percutaneous discectomy and chemonucleolysis.

Although in certain centers percutaneous discectomy is being utilized for the treatment of lumbago and discogenic pain [14], in the United States we have adhered to the criteria originally developed by the Human Experimentation Committee of The Graduate Hospital in affiliation with the University of Pennsylvania School of Medicine [7, 9].

All of our patients presented persistent sciatic pain and had failed to respond to a reasonable course of conservative therapy. All had one or two neurological deficits. In the absence of neurological deficits, we looked for a positive correlative electromyographic evaluation. Their tension signs, such as the straight leg raising test, Lasègue or sitting root pain, were positive. Finally, all had a positive correlative myelogram or positive CT and MRI studies.

In recent years, we have been able to depend on the combination of a CT and MRI studies for the localization of the symptom-producing discs. This has eliminated the need for myelographic studies on a routine basis.

The role of conservative therapy for the management of radicular pain due to a protruded disc, should not be ignored. The majority of these patients do respond to well-planned conservative therapy. Such treatment should include bed rest, non-steroidal anti-inflammatory drugs or short-term steroid therapy. Educational programs, physical therapy, exercises and perhaps, manipulation treatment. However, one should not get locked into prolonged and unreasonable conservative management. Symptoms associated with intra- and perineural fibrosis, secondary to protracted mechanical pressure to the nerve root may be irreversible. The progression or development of a neurological deficit necessitates the consideration for surgical decompression. Finally, the patient's level of pain tolerance and the demand for the use of narcotic-based medication should effect the timing for the surgical intervention.

The rehabilitation of a drug-dependent patient may be much more complicated than the slim chance of a surgical mishap.

As far as the type of herniation is concerned, we have treated both central and lateral herniations successfully through the percutaneous approach. The size of the herniation also should not be a major concern. We have decompressed and partially evacuated rather large contained subligamentous fragments. The proper positioning of the sheath is of particular importance for the evacuation of the latter herniations. Sequestrated discs, previously operated discs, failed chemonucleolysis, spinal stenosis and cauda equina syndrome are not candidates for percutaneous discectomy.

Operative Technique

Our arsenal of instrumentation has been growing rapidly. The original instrumentation is still being utilized, which consists of an 18-gauge spinal needle, a Kirschner wire, various sizes of cannulated trocars and sheaths, cutting instruments, forceps, curets, deflector tube and goniometer. Powered tools and scopes are also available. Recently, we have been experimenting with a working scope which allows a uniportal approach to the intervertebral disc. The tip of the flexible instruments or the laser probe is easily maneuvered in the course of the surgical procedure. Our operative technique and instrumentation has been published in detail [7, 9]; however, the highlights of this operation and important points of consideration are as follows.

To diminish the chance of infection and its serious consequences, we strongly feel that the percutaneous discectomy should be performed in the operating room in a strictly sterile environment. We use a prophylactic antibiotic for 24 h in all of our patients. Patients are placed on a radiolucent adjustable frame, which allows the freedom of the abdomen and flattens the lumbosacral angle.

The proper positioning is of particular importance for L 5 – S 1 disc extraction.

The procedure must be performed under local anesthesia. The intraoperative communication with the patient is essential.

The correct positioning of the needle is the most important single step which will ultimately affect the final outcome of this operative procedure. The angle of introduction of the needle may be predetermined by an abdominal CT exposed through the herniated intervertebral disc.

The inserted needle should penetrate the sacrospinalis, quadratus lumborsum and psoas major muscles in its path [6].

When the needle is introduced lateral to the boundary of these muscles, there will be a greater likelihood of entrance into the abdominal cavity, causing serious complications.

In contrast, entry too close to the midline effects the adequate evacuation.

The tip of the needle should enter the annulus just lateral to the proximal articular process of the inferior vertebra. This position is visualized at 1 or 11 o'clock in the lateral x-ray projection. In the AP projection, the tip of the needle is seen in alignment or just lateral to the mid-portion of the pedicle (Fig. 1).

The utilization of the cannulated trocar (Fig. 2) allows the precise insertion of the instruments and reduces the chance of neural injury or the development of periannular bleeding and psoas hematoma.

To maintain the intradiscal pressure at a reduced level following the surgery, adequate annular fenestration is desirable.

The working sheath is then introduced. The design of the instruments permits only a 2 cm penetration of the forceps and curet in the disc space. However, if a deeper penetration is desirable, one can engage and advance the sheath into the annular fibers.

The evacuation of the disc material is achieved with straight, angled, flexible forceps, curets and power tools. We are performing all of our discectomies

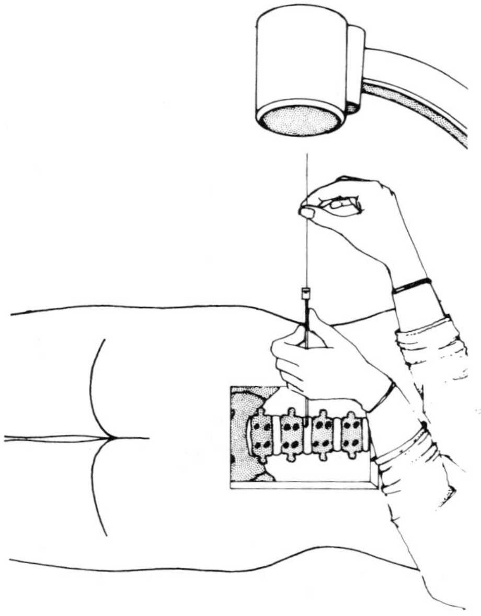

Fig. 1. Correct position of needle in AP x-ray projection and insertion of Kirschner wire

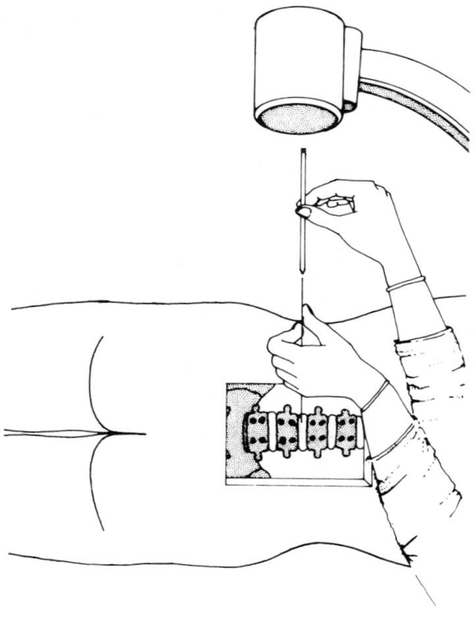

Fig. 2. The introduction of cannulated trocar over the Kirschner wire

through a uniportal approach; however, we have used the biportal approach to achieve interbody arthrodesis (Figs. 3, 4).

The ultrasound and laser beam also can be used for this endeavor; however, their usefulness at the current state of knowledge remains questionable.

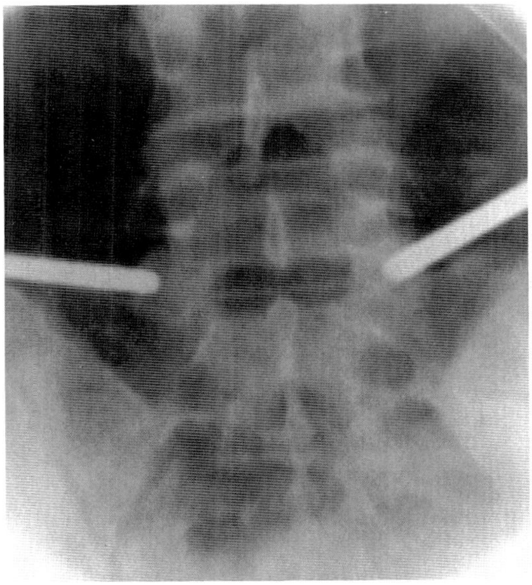

Fig. 3. Interoperative x-ray, biportal approach to L5–S1 disc space

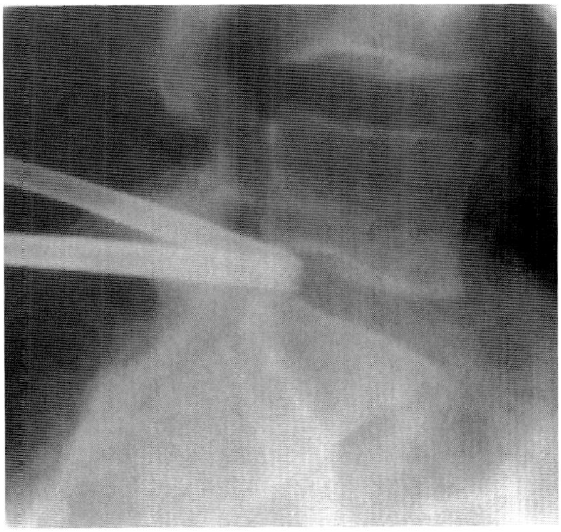

Fig. 4. Lateral view of biportal approach

Results

A prospective study of 100 patients with sciatic pain who were treated by percutaneous discectomy was recently completed at The Graduate Hospital [10]. Ninety-two (92) of these patients had a positive correlative myelography and CT scan studies.

In eight (8) patients, only CT and MRI studies were done. Most of our patients were admitted to the hospital a day prior to the surgery for a myelogram and a general medical evaluation. These patients were discharged approximately 24 h following their surgical procedure. The average postoperative stay in the hospital was 2 days. This statistic included the patients who were kept in the hospital for a longer period of time in earlier years, when we were gaining experience in this operative procedure. All of these patients are up and about following their surgery. Certainly, this operation can be performed on an Out-Patient basis.

The average nuclear material extracted was 1.91 g. The follow-up period was 1 to 6 years and the majority of them had greater than 2 years of postoperative observation.

Utilizing modified MacNab criteria, questionnaires, personal interviews and physical examinations, 87% of procedures were judged to be a success. Twelve patients failed percutaneous lumbar discectomy and 11 of them subsequently required laminectomy.

The failures were attributed to undiagnosed sequestration, degenerative spondylolisthesis, lateral stenosis, inadequate evacuation, drug dependency and psychological disorders.

In response to the self-assessment questionnaires, 65% considered themselves to be cured while 35% felt that the PLD had helped them.

We have not encountered any serious complications such as neurovascular injuries or infections.

Conclusion

The percutaneous lumbar discectomy, in our hands, has proven to be non-destructive, safe, effective and cost-efficient [2, 4]. The earlier concern regarding intraoperative complications, namely the development of neural injury, seems to be unfounded.

The success of percutaneous lumbar discectomy hinges on the following principle:

- Knowledge of the anatomy of the spinal nerve and its surrounding structures
- Adherence to the detail of the operative technique
- Careful isolation of the symptom-producing disc
- Sufficient evacuation of both central and peripheral nuclear fragments and adequate annular fenestration
- Proper patient selection and recognition of the effect of psychological factors on the persistence of pain syndrome remains the single and most important factor effecting the final outcome of percutaneous lumbar discectomy.

References

1. Hult L (1951) Retroperitoneal disc fenestration in low back pain and sciatica. Acta Orthop Scand 20: 342
2. Kambin P (1985) Percutaneous lateral discectomy. Journal of Orthopaedics Today, February 1985
3. Kambin P (1987) Bulging annulus. Orthopaedic Transactions, Vol. II, Number 1, Spring 1987
4. Kambin P (1988) Percutaneous lumbar discectomy – Safe, effective and cost-efficient. Orthopaedics Today, February 1988
5. Kambin P (in press) Percutaneous lumbar discectomy current practice. Surgical Round for Orthopaedics
6. Kambin P, Brager M (1987) Percutaneous posterolateral discectomy: Anatomy and mechanism. Clin Orthop 223: 145
7. Kambin P, Gellman H (1983) Percutaneous lateral discectomy of the lumbar spine: A preliminary report. Clin Orthop 174: 127–132
8. Kambin P, Sampson S (1984) Laminectomy versus percutaneous lateral discectomy: A comparative study. Orthop Trans 8: 408
9. Kambin P, Sampson S (1986) Posterolateral percutaneous suction-excision of herniated lumbar intervertebral discs: Report of interim results. Clin Orthop 207: 37
10. Kambin P, Schaffer JL (in press) Percutaneous lumbar discectomy: prospective review of 100 patients. Clin Orthop and Related Research
11. Kambin P, Nixon JE, Chait A (in press) Bulging annulus pathophysiology and roentgenographic findings. Spine
12. McCulloch JA (1980) Chemonucleolysis. Experience with 2000 cases. Clin Orthop and Related Research 146: 128
13. Mixter WJ, Barr JS (1934) Rupture of intervertebral disc with involvement of the spinal canal. N Engl J Med 211: 210
14. Monteiro A (1987) Lateral hole decompression of the lumbar spine. Presented at the Internat'l. Symposium on Percutaneous Lumbar Discectomy. Philadelphia, November 6–7, 1987
15. Smith L (1963) Enzyme dissolution of the intervertebral disc. Nature 4887: 198
16. Stern I, Smith L (1967) Dissolution by chymopapain in vitro of tissue from normal or prolapsed intervertebral discs. Clin. Orthop. 50: 269

Indication and Technique of Percutaneous Nucleotomy with Discoscopy – Eight Years Experience (1979–1987)

A. Schreiber, Y. Suezawa, and H. Leu [1]

Introduction

Since the original description of the technique of open hemilaminotomy with discotomy [6], orthopedic surgeons have encountered postoperative problems of local epidural cicatrization, segmental problems by induced instability, and dorsal interarticular incongruency: the so-called posthemilaminotomy syndrome. While this classic open procedure allows good exposure of the local disc herniation, the surgical approach interferes directly with the main dorsal stabilizing muscles and ligament structures. Aware of these disadvantages, several other possibilities were tested and described in the early fifties. For instance Hult [4] introduced the purely retroperitoneal disc fenestration; the method was abandoned, however, because of the instrumental problems encountered to effect sufficient removal of the dorsal annulus fibrosus.

Evolution of the Technical Procedure

In the purely diagnostic field, the dorsolateral puncture of the intervertebral space was mentioned in 1934 by Ball and further described in 1956 by Craig [2]. In the early seventies, Kambin [5] applied a modified Craig instrumentarium for minimum possible fenestration of the annulus fibrosus, this still in combination with the classical dorsolateral open hemilaminotomy.

In the same period, Hijikata developed and applied new instruments for closed percutaneous therapeutic removal of disc herniations by dorsolateral intervertebral puncture. His original publication dates from 1975 [3].

In our clinic, we adapted this operative technique in 1979 using Hijikata's original instruments. Soon we recognized that this instrument, conceived for the small Asian build, could not satisfy the needs for the bigger European stature. So, in cooperation with our biomechanical department, we redesigned and adapted the tools in 1980. This pluri-cannular instrument is now in use after several further modifications in design and material (Fig. 1).

[1] Department of Orthopaedic Surgery, Balgrist, Medical School, University of Zürich, Forchstrasse 340, 8008 Zürich, Switzerland

Percutaneous Lumbar Discectomy
Ed. by H. M. Mayer and M. Brock

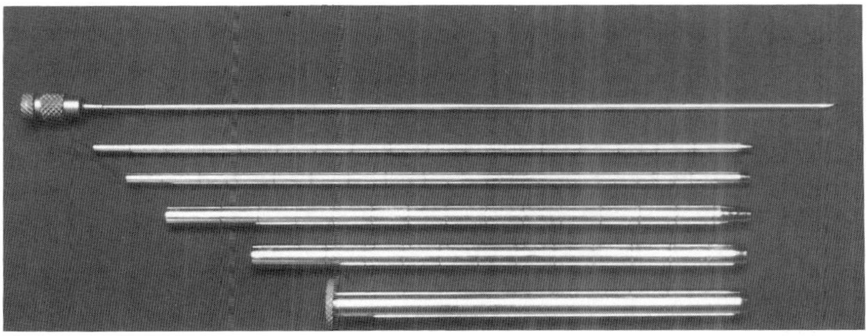

Fig. 1. The original "Balgrist cannula set" (Howmedica®) consists of a double-walled guide-needle (top) and a line of telescopically superimposable cannulas with the big working cannula of internal diameter 7.5 mm

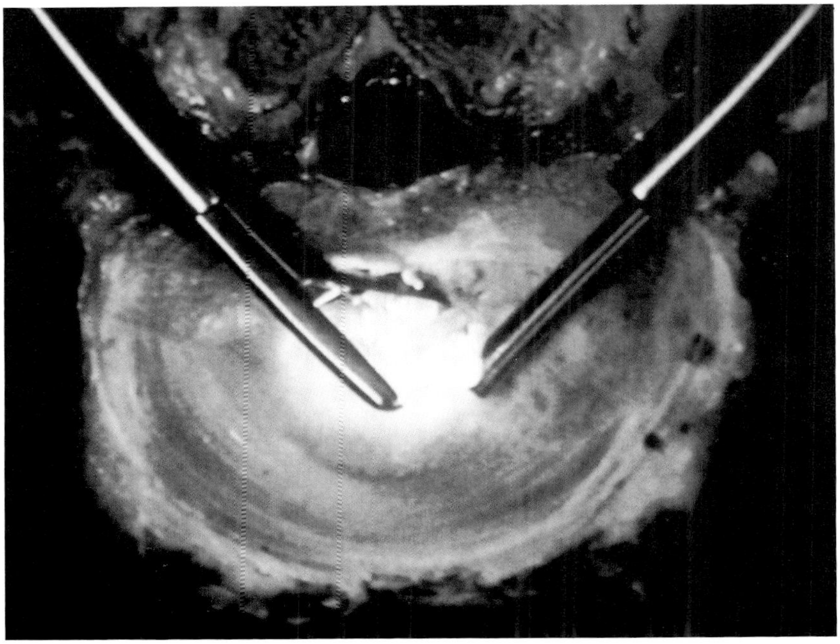

Fig. 2. Percutaneous discoscopy allows direct vision control of the dorsolateral percutaneous discotomy from both sides

During the early years of using this technique, we encountered a few cases in which we could not obtain a satisfactory removal of the subligamentous herniation, even when entering from both sides. It was not possible to really locate the dislodged disc material, especially in the posterior subligamentous area, and extract it precisely. Theoretically, better control could be done by permanent fluoroscopic observation, but such an amount of x-ray exposure was obviously not permissible.

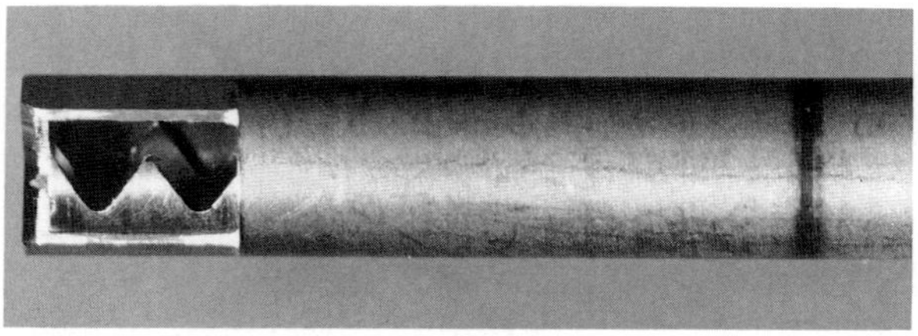

Fig. 3. The design of shaver heads depends crucially on their use: this model with apicolateral aperture and serrated rotating blade is especially useful in disintegrating bigger intradiscal fragments, also laterally to the cannula axis

Experiments on cadaver specimens in our laboratory demonstrated in 1981 that the former experimental technique of myeloscopy, described by Burman [1], Pool [9] and Ooi [8], could be adapted also for intradiscal optical control. Thus in 1982 [10, 16, 17], with the correspondingly modified optical device, we performed successfully, for the first time "in vivo", this procedure which we call "percutaneous discoscopy" (Fig. 2).

In 1985 Onik [7] reported the successful application of an adapted motorized shaver in the percutaneous procedure. In our clinic, since early 1986, we have employed a modified arthroscopy shaver with adapted working heads in combination with suction and irrigation (Fig. 3). By means of the shaver we can disintegrate bigger discal fragments before extracting them, and also wash out small particles left behind by the forceps. The principle of permanent irrigation also diminishes the risk of bacteriological contamination in this bradytrophic area.

The technical evolution of shaver design is continuing; with appropriate head design, precise preparation of the adjacent vertebral plates also became possible. This will be the first precondition to fulfil in cases where we attempt to perform intervertebral bony fusion.

Principles of Indication for Percutaneous Nucleotomy

In comparison to other concurrent operative technique of lumbar disc surgery, the spectrum of application of percutaneous nucleotomy has widened with growing experience. Today we limit the indication for chemonucleolysis to rare cases with insufficiently accessible level L 5/S 1 [11]. Beside the recurrent problems of allergic reactions to chymopapain, we found considerably less relief of low back pain even though the comparable effect on sciatica was about the same. In the field of open operative procedures, the spectrum of indications has correspondingly been reduced by the new technique of percutaneous nucleotomy, which is less invasive [12, 13, 15]. The actual spectrum of our indications for different techniques in lumbar disc surgery is shown in Table 1.

The indication for percutaneous nucleotomy with discoscopy is very broad. The limits in the fields of slight disc protrusion or the considerable subligamentous herniation are still in evolution. Relative prospective studies are in progress.

Percutaneous nucleotomy covers today the unsuccessfully treated sciaticas. We must accept a period of three or even six months to observe the success of conservative treatment and we ought to take advantages of any conservative

Table 1. Spectrum of indications in lumbar disc surgery

	radicular symptoms	
disc protrusion bulging disc	subligamentous disc herniation	sequestration mass herniation
	<------ conventional open discotomy	----->
	<– chemonucleolysis – >	
>> – <––– Percutaneous discotomy	–––––––––––––	> – <<

Table 2. PN: indications versus contraindications

Indications	Contraindications
– disc-protrusion	– hernia with sequester
– subligamentous herniation	– mass prolapse in myelography
– spondylolysis/-olisthesis	– severe neurological deficiency
– narrow spinal canal	– aggressive osteochondrosis
– recurrent disc herniation	

procedure to profit by the chance of nonoperative healing. The period of such treatment will depend also on the structural disc pathology as described later under preoperative radiologic screening.

In our experience, the PN procedure offers valuable possibilities, especially in patients whose discogenous sciatica is added to another preexisting structural deficiency, such as discontinuity of the dorsal pediculo-articular pillar (Table 2). In these cases, any further destabilization of musculoligamentous structures by an open operative approach may favor clinical decompensation with a subjectively poor clinical outcome, due to developing non-discogenous symptoms postoperatively.

The symptomatic narrow spinal canal, in most cases primarily due to a combination of bony formation, progressive arthritic deformation and additional disc protrusion, represents also one of the favorite indications for percutaneous nucleotomy: removal of the often critically limiting disc component by the PN procedure. We can therefore obtain the required decompression without causing persisting epidural cicatrization. The generally less stressful percutaneous intervention can also be applied in elderly patients.

The indication in recurrent disc herniation after previous surgical procedures is based on similar principles: the PN technique does not induce epidural cicatrization any more and spares already impaired dorsal stabilizing structures. Obviously, the other general evaluation criteria for the indication of percutaneous nucleotomy have to be considered.

The list of strict contraindications is also shown in Table 2. Suspicion of free sequestration into the spinal canal prohibits the PN procedure. Any blind extraction of free sequesters out of the epidural space remains too precarious; even with direct discoscopic guidance we cannot control any "fishing" beyond the dorsal longitudinal ligament without risking damage to the contents of the spinal canal. At the moment, no available technique of supplementary myeloscopic control can yet reduce this problem appreciably.

The contraindication of subligamentous mass prolapse for percutaneous removal is given for three reasons:

- it can be difficult to distinguish partial sequestration from strictly subligamentous mass prolapse in radiologic screening.
- the extraction of bulky subligamentous masses toward the intervertebral space can be mechanically impossible.
- in cases with concomitant epidural cicatrization, some unpredictable risk of a distraction rupture of thinned dorsal ligament or of the dural convolute could occur.

Cases with severe neurological deficiencies, such as rapidly increasing sensomotoric radicular failure with considerable herniation evident on a CT scan, still remain an indication for immediate open operative removal. In such situations, apart from the possible waste of time, there may be a certain risk due to complementary invasive diagnostic investigations, e.g., by raising the intradiscal pressure further while conducting the otherwise valuable discography.

The presence of active osteochondrotic alterations, besides a respective discogenous narrowing of the spinal canal, forms another contraindication for percutaneous nucleotomy. Even if good local decompression of the spinal canal can be obtained, the osteochondrotic process itself will continue with all its implications. We therefore think that, in such cases, a radical discectomy with following intervertebral fusion ought to be done. Theoretically this combined procedure could be realized also via a percutaneous approach. For the moment, some technical difficulties in preparing the adjacent vertebral plates still have to be solved. Even though this procedure is still not standardized, early experience encourages us to push in this direction.

Preoperative Screening

In spite of all imaging investigations, obviously clinical orthopedic and neurologic examination remains indispensable. In cases with contradictory senso-motoric signs, a supplementary electromyography allows better segmental determination. Quantitative measuring of disc degeneration by discomanometry can further help to class different prospective groups. The preoperative radiologic screening follows the scheme shown in Table 3.

Obviously all non-invasive investigations have to be applied first. Whenever the CT scan cannot give a strictly direct correlation to the clinical signs, we still use lumbar myelography. In our experience, myelography, by using modern water-soluble contrast media, has become well tolerable and can give a precise analysis of the sagittal dura borderlines in their continuity, and this also in different functional positions. So the relative measurement of segmental disc protrusion can be directly compared in relation to the previous axial CT scan. The

Table 3. Preoperative radiologic screening

Imaging technique	Main check
1. biplane standard x-ray	bone status, arthritic changes intervertebral height
2. computed tomography	dorsal disc border, width of spinal canal
3. myelography	qualitative CSF testing dural/radicular borders protrusion/hernia comparing functional positions/levels
+ following CT scan	epidural cicatrization root configuration
4. discography + following CT scan	dorsal density of annulus fibrosus dorsolateral disc border dorsal density (extension of degeneration)
5. magnetic resonance imaging	sagittal/transversal analysis in various directions histometabolic activity

different rotary positions also allow comparison of functional bulging at different levels.

In static sagittal evaluation, magnetic resonance imaging can concur to the myelography; its main value lies in screening also the histometabolic activity with its large differential diagnosis. The main practical problems, even today, are its restricted availability and the still impossible control under different functional positions.

The CT scan with additional contrast media can also be easily combined with myelography. This technique allows one especially to distinguish between disc pathology and/or cicatrizations, particularly in recurrent herniation.

Only the now routinely performed discography can answer the question whether the annulus fibrosus forms a tight union with the dorsal longitudinal ligament or whether there is a discontinuity, which might even include a sequestration (Fig. 4). In inconsistent findings with native CT and myelography, the discography can be immediately followed by further CT scan [14]. This "discoscan" allows evaluation of the character of disc degeneration and especially of the dorsolateral and lateral disc border. Moreover, it shows precisely the localization of any dorsal leak at the annulus/ligament border.

The Balgrist PN-Procedure with Discoscopy Today

In the operation theater, the patient is placed in a prone position with slight flexion in the hips. Percutaneous nucleotomy can be performed in local anesthesia, especially at the level of L4/5 or above. In the lumbosacral transition with individually variable anatomic properties, as well as in bi-level percutaneous approach, a general anesthesia may be preferred by the patient.

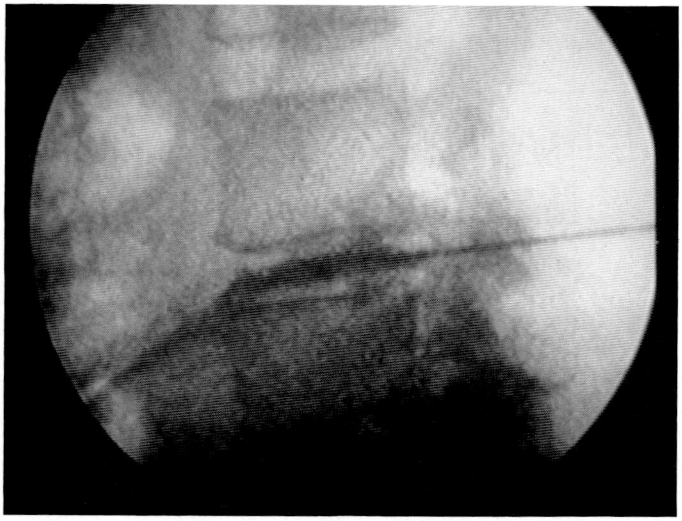

Fig. 4. The discography, now routinely performed as first step of the PN operation procedure, has to confirm an intact dorsal annulus fibrosus. In this case (female, born 1963, reg. no. 312967) beside the subligamentous protrusion there is a relatively undegenerated disc: the contrast medium remains locally concentrated

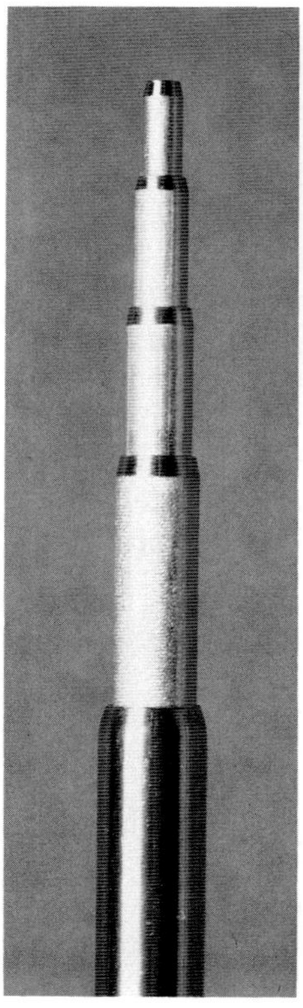

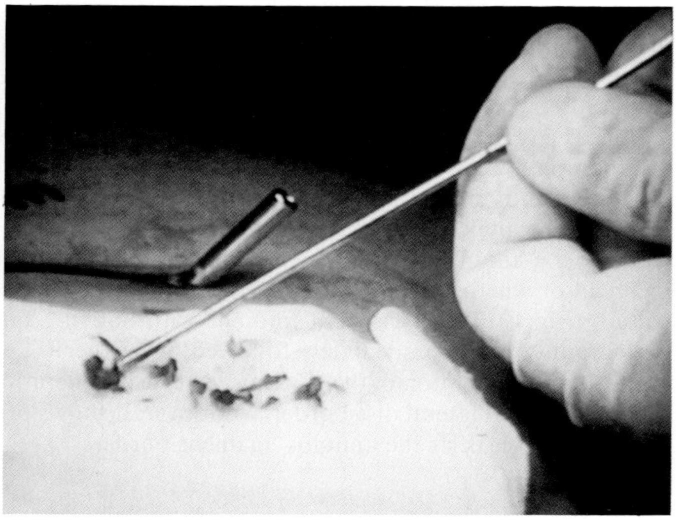

Fig. 6. Operation site: the disc protrusion is removed by extracting the disc material in the dorsal area by different tools under direct discoscopic control, here, for example, by the smaller forceps of outer diameter 3.5 mm

◀ **Fig. 5.** Because the tip is conical, the soft tissues are gradually penetrated by the superimposable cannulas without direct cutting. This principle also prevents the risk of radicular nerve damage

The cannular set for percutaneous nucleotomy contains a double-walled guide needle and a set of telescopically superimposable cannulas with the big working cannula having an internal diameter of 7.5 mm. The guide needle, introduced first through a dorsolateral approach, whose entry distance to the midline has been measured on the CT scan, is positioned under fluoroscopic control in the center of the nucleus pulposus. This needle represents the central axis of the later working lumen of the biggest cannula and serves to directly perform the discography. Under local anesthesia, it is possible to perform also the provocation test: a positive "memory pain" confirms the local discogenous origin of the sciatica.

Each cannula is conical at its tip; in this way the soft tissues can be gradually penetrated without cutting (Fig. 5). After the positioning of the third cannula, a first portion of disc material is brought out from the nucleus by the smallest forceps. This prevents further raising of intradiscal pressure and facilitates penetration of the remaining two big cannulas. By means of the working cannula, further disc material is brought out by forceps and different shaver models, as mentioned above (Fig. 6). To obtain a second percutaneous approach, the same cannular instruments are brought in from the opposite side.

Through the rigid optical lenses in combination with a chip camera and high-resolution color monitor, the intradiscal removal can be controlled directly from the opposite side (Figs. 7, 8). By superimposing a sketch transparency showing various available optical configurations onto the CT scan, we check preoperatively which of the optical tools will be the most suitable to carry out the percutaneous procedure. In most cases, an optic of 90 degrees of view with a deflection of 70 degrees will be the right one. By this optically guided discharge procedure, we can precisely point and remove also major subligamentous herniations. It is not seldom possible to extract subligamentous herniations of considerable size in this manner.

While in the early years we always attempted to remove as much disc material as possible, we now try to remove only the most we can get in the dorsal subligamentous part of the disc. In the more frontal disc area we try to remove whatever is loose and fragmented portions that could be subject to later dorsal displacement. We believe this is better to prevent bulging and, furthermore, even collapsing disc by maintaining an antero-posterior bridge that can bear axial load.

Postoperative mobilization is effected on the first postoperative day with an elastic abdominal bandage. The physiotherapeutic program is strictly limited to isometric stabilizing exercises in the first month following percutaneous nucleotomy. Dismission from hospital is usually possible four to ten days after the intervention. This intensively controlled primary rehabilitation phase helps to prevent muscular imbalance during early mobilization. After four to six weeks, the rehabilitation program provides controlled lumbar mobilization. The patients get back to work between six and ten weeks postoperatively, depending on the type of occupation.

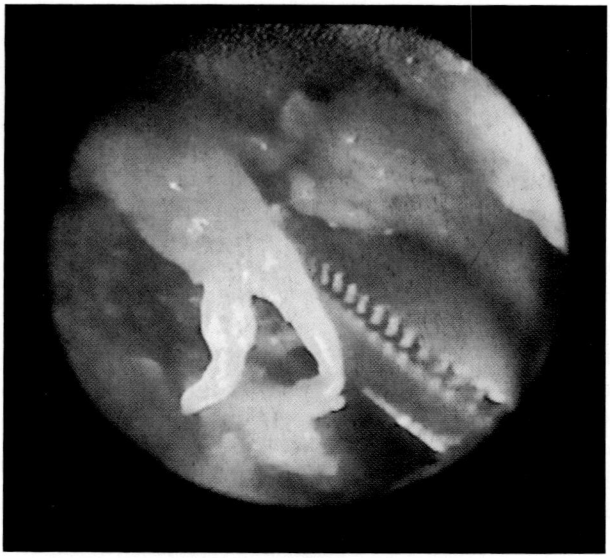

Fig. 7. Under discoscopic control, disc material can be precisely targeted and removed: here a serrated forceps is introduced under discoscopic control

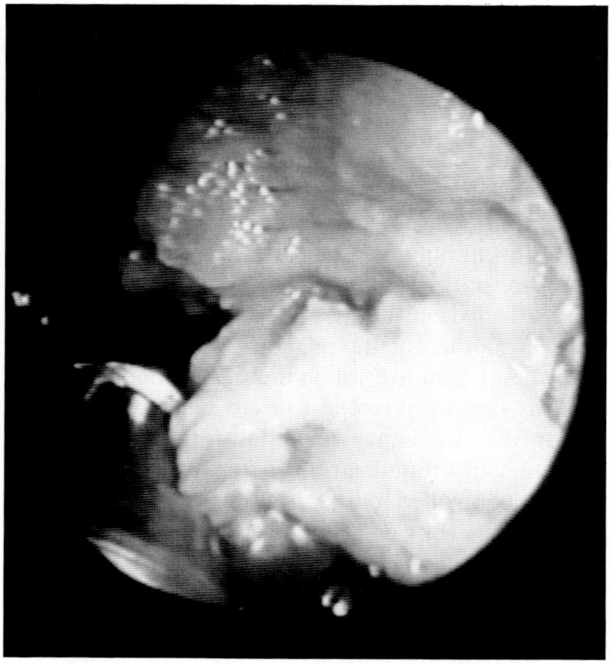

Fig. 8. The also discoscopically controlled shaver disintegrates large disc fragments and brings out small fragments left behind by the forceps

Practical Experience and Results

Between 1979 and the end of 1987 we treated 109 patients (68 m, 41 f) with percutaneous nucleotomy in our clinic. The annual statistic shows a markedly increasing number in the last years. The age at operation ranged from 19 to 71 years, with an average of about 39 years. The average follow-up in this report was near 2¾ years. The operated discs were at more than one level in twenty cases (Table 4).

In 48/109 cases there were isolated disc protrusions/herniations without simultaneous low back pathology. These patients constitute group 1. In 61/109 cases, there were simultaneous alterations such as narrow spinal canal, spondylolysis/olisthesis or recurrent disc pathology after open operative procedure. These patients make up group 2. The follow-up results (Table 5) were classified according to the Balgrist nucleotomy score [13].

A very good, good or fair result was obtained in 79 of the 109 patients (72.5%). The corresponding percentage in Group 1 was 75% and, remarkably, 70% in Group 2 (Table 6). These results of percutaneous nucleotomy are in

Table 4. 128 PN-operated disc levels in 109 patients: the most treated segment was at L 4/5; even when sometimes difficult, nearly every fifth case was successfully operated at level L 5/S 1, also with percutaneous nucleotomy

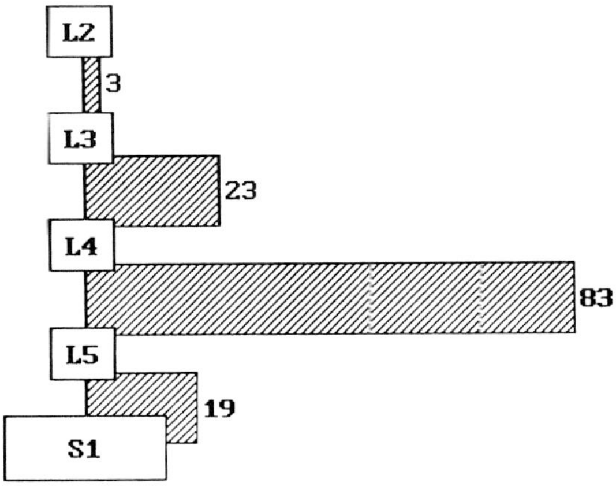

Table 5. The Balgrist score criteria for nucleotomy

Criteria	Description
1. pain:	ischialgia, lumbago, drug requirements
2. spinal weight bearing:	sitting/standing/walking, ±corset requirement
3. spinal mobility:	finger-floor distance, reactive scoliosis
4. neurological signs:	radicular signs, sensomotor damages
5. rehabilitation:	professional reintegration, hobby/sport

Table 6. Results (n = 109) in Balgrist score assessment

Assessment	group 1 (n = 48)	group 2 (n = 61)	group 1 + 2 (n = 109)
very good – fair	75%	70%	72.2%
poor	25%	30%	27.8%

contrast with a series of follow-up on 283 patients from our clinic after classical open disc surgery, where the favorable results of the analog Group 1 reached a similar 74%, but in Group 2 did not exceed 31%.

The difficulties and complications encountered have to be separated into three classes: the first is failure due to insufficient operative decompression, the seond is failure due to technical intraoperative complications, and the third class because of unexpected reactive alterations after an adequate operative procedure.

Thus in 10 cases, we observed insufficient removal of the discogenous narrowing in postoperative CT or myelographic checks. In 9 of these cases, already during operation, it was evident that the mass of herniated disc material had been underestimated in the preoperative screening, or a sequestration had been missed.

As a direct technical complication, we have to report an accidental puncture of the A. sigmoidea by the guide needle. Unfortunately the outer guide, blocked by bending of the tube, was pushed too far forward while overslipped by the tube of next caliber. The silent bleeding was discovered within six hours after nucleotomy and was managed by a ventrolateral abdominal approach. The results of the percutaneous discotomy in this case today are good. The material of the guide needle has since been modified so that accidental bending is less possible.

As neurological complications, we encountered two transient irritations of the lumbar plexus due to local hematoma after a missed percutaneous approach to the level L 5/S 1.

In another 8 patients, there were signs of postoperative osteochondritis in the first three to six months. A local bacterial genesis was proved in only one of these cases. This one, and a second patient with aseptic osteochondritis, had to be treated by dorsolateral spondylotomy. In the other cases, radiologic alterations were quite impressive, but other inflammatory parameters such as ^{Tc}scintigraphy or hematologic alterations were not present. Nevertheless, magnetic resonance imaging showed, in one case, an early inflammatory process with propagation across the adjacent vertebral plates. The symptoms were successfully treated with a temporary corset and antiphlogistics, and therefore we could not verify the histological site.

Having seen some similar cases of focal circumscribed osteolysis with transient low back pain of lesser degree, we think that these alterations may be due to accidental scraping of adjacent vertebral plates with subsequent direct reaction of the underlying cancellous bone to degradation metabolites in the evacuated disc space.

Discussion

The follow-up results of this series of 109 patients treated with percutaneous nucleotomy from 1979 to end of 1987 have been found satisfactory to very good in more than 70% of cases. We have to underline especially the relative favorable results of percutaneous nucleotomy in our group 2 with simultaneous low back pathology in comparison to the results of our control series after open hemilaminotomy/discotomy. This proves the value of the sparing percutaneous approach, also in cases with simultaneous risk of musculoligamentous decompensation.

The reoperation rate, over 50% until 1980, has decreased to under 20% at the end of 1987. As shown above, most of the failures has been due to inappropriate preoperative diagnostics such as an omitted sequester or underestimated subligamentous mass prolapse. Newer preoperative screening, e.g. with contrast-aided myelo-CT or disco-scan, have decreased the failure rate in our later series. Supplementary quantitative evaluation of disc degeneration, e.g. discomanometric preoperative evaluation, has to be continued to contribute to further standardized indication also of percutaneous nucleotomy. On the other hand, a more refined operative technique with pointed subligamentous discharge and use of continuously modified instruments will help to obtain even better results.

Early experience with intervertebral bone grafting also indicates a great therapeutic potential in the percutaneous treatment of segmental instability. The aim may be not to effect primarily intervertebral fusion, but instead to maintain intervertebral height by means of an intradiscal space holder. Whether this can also be a percutaneous allograft is a matter of further research.

References

1. Burman MS (1931) Myeloscopy or the direct visualisation of spinal cord. J Bone Joint Surg 13:695–696
2. Craig FS (1956) Vertebral body biopsy. J Bone Joint Surg 38A:93–95
3. Hijikata S (1975) Percutane Nucleotomie – neue Behandlung der Discushernie. J Toden Hosp 5:39
4. Hult L (1951) Retroperitoneal disc fenestration in low back pain and sciatica. Acta Orthop Scand 20:342
5. Kambin P, Gellman H (1983) Percutaneous lateral discectomy of the lumbar spine. A preliminary report. Clin Orthop 174:127
6. Mixter WJ, Barr JS (1934) Rupture of the intervertebral disc with involvement of the spinal canal. N Engl J Med 211:210–215
7. Onik G, Helms CA, Ginsburg L, Hoaglund FT, Morris J (1985) Percutaneous lumbar discectomy using a new aspiration probe. AJNR 6:290
8. Ooi Y, Satoh Y, Sugawara S, Mikanagi K, Morisaki N (1977) Myeloscopy. Internat Orthop (SICOT) 1:107–111
9. Pool JL (1938) Myeloscopy, diagnostic inspection of the cauda equina by means of an endoscope. Bull Neurol Inst 7:178–139
10. Schreiber A, Suezawa Y (1986) Transdiscoscopic percutaneous nucleotomy in disc herniation. Orthop Rev 15:75

11. Schreiber A, Suezawa Y, Jacob HAC (1987) Indications et technique de la nucléotomie percutanée et de la chimionucléolyse. S.O.F.C.O.T. 1986. Rev Chir Orthop Suppl-II: 73
12. Schreiber A, Suezawa Y, Leu HJ (1988) Therapie des Bandscheibenprolaps: Chemonukleolyse versus perkutane Nukleotomie. DMW (in print)
13. Schreiber A, Suezawa Y, Leu HJ (1988) Does percutaneous nucleotomy with discoscopy replace conventional discotomy? Clin Orthop (in print)
14. Shigehiko I (1988) CT-assisted discography. J Jpn Orthop Assoc 62: 345–358
15. Suezawa Y (1982) Kreuzschmerzen in der Orthopädie – Heutiger Stand ihrer Therapien. Schweiz Rundschau Med (Praxis) 71: 783
16. Suezawa Y, Schreiber A (1988) Perkutane Nukleotomie mit Diskoskopie: 7-jährige Erfahrung und Ergebnisse. Z Orthop 126: 1–7
17. Suezawa Y, Jacob HAC, Brandenberg JE, Blasbalg DT (1983) Diskoskopie – ein weiterer Schritt zur Diagnostik und Behandlung der lumbalen Diskusläsion. In: von Hackenbroch MH (ed) Biomechanik der Wirbelsäule. Georg Thieme, Stuttgart, pp 130

Percutaneous Lumbar Discectomy – The Berlin Technique

H.M. Mayer and M. Brock [1]

Introduction

Various techniques of percutaneous lumbar discectomy have been described since 1975 [1, 2, 4, 7, 16, 17]. However, since surgical goals and pathophysiological conceptions of the effects of these procedures differ quite considerably [3, 5, 7, 13–15], we feel compelled to define and review the current procedures before describing our own technique.

In *percutaneous lumbar discectomy* (*PLD*), the herniated nucleus pulposus is removed by means of rigid forceps (straight or angled) as well as flexible forceps [5]. Automated shaver systems, known from arthroscopic surgery, accelerate and improve this procedure [15, 17, 18]. A *partial or total nucleectomy* is thereby achieved, resulting in "open" decompression of the intervertebral space, since the center of the disc is reached through a hole in the annulus fibrosus.

In *percutaneous lumbar discectomy with discoscopy*, a second (contralateral) approach permits *selective nucleectomy* under visual control [15, 18]. In *automated percutaneous lumbar discectomy* (*APLD*), a disposable "nucleotome probe" leads to closed *internal decompression* of the disc space by removal of the central parts of the nucleus pulposus. Selective nucleectomy, e.g. the removal of subligamentous prolapses, is not possible. The therapeutic effect is comparable to that achieved by chemonucleolysis.

Instruments

Visually controlled selective percutaneous nucleectomy should be performed with instruments that meet the standards for surgical efficacy and patient safety [8]. The instruments required for percutaneous access comprise an 18G cannula (for deep local anesthesia, puncturing the disc and discography), a round-tipped guide wire, a blunt obturator with a central hollow and working tubes with inner diameters ranging from 4.6 to 7.5 mm (Figs. 1 and 2). Various annulus trephines (Fig. 3), rigid (straight or angled) as well as flexible forceps which can be directed through a deflector tube have been developed for perforating the annulus fibrosus

[1] Neurochirurgische Klinik, Klinikum Steglitz, Freie Universität Berlin, Hindenburgdamm 30, 1000 Berlin 45, FRG

Percutaneous Lumbar Discectomy
Ed. by H.M. Mayer and M. Brock

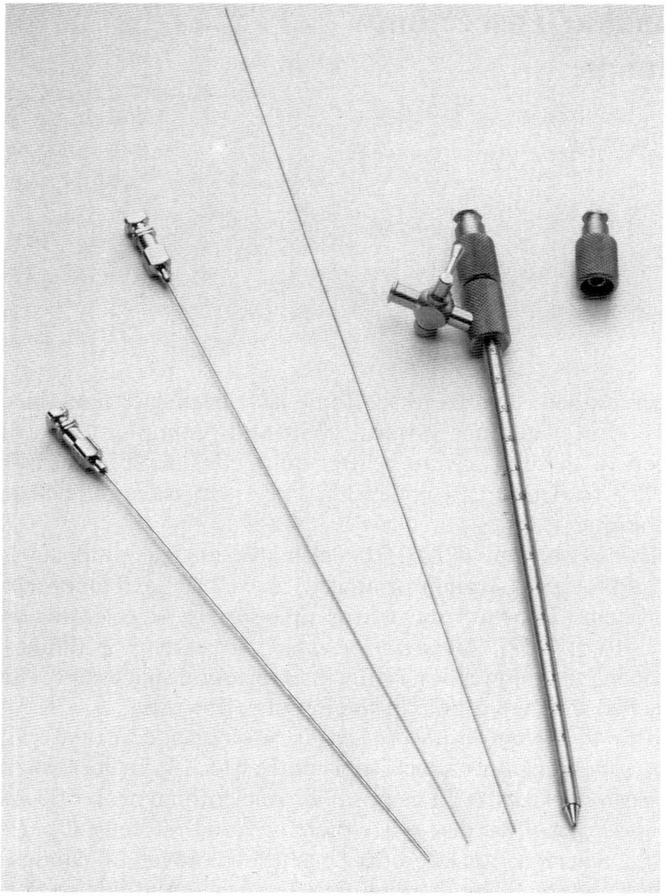

Fig. 1. Cannula, guide wire, obturator and working sleeve for percutaneous access (with kind permission of Aesculap Werke AG, Tuttlingen, FRG)

and for selective removal of herniated nucleus pulposus. To reach the critical dorsal and dorsolateral parts of the intervertebral space, a wide-range deflector which permits angulating a flexible forceps has been developed (Fig. 4).

Modified shavers and cutters which reach sites beyond the working range of manual instruments have proved their efficacy (Figs. 5a–c). However, these instruments are fully functional only when coupled to a high-powered suction apparatus such as the ones used for abdominal lipectomy in plastic surgery (Fig. 6). Intermittent visual control of percutaneous discectomy is possible with a wide-angle discoscope coupled to a CCD endoscopic camera system (Fig. 7).

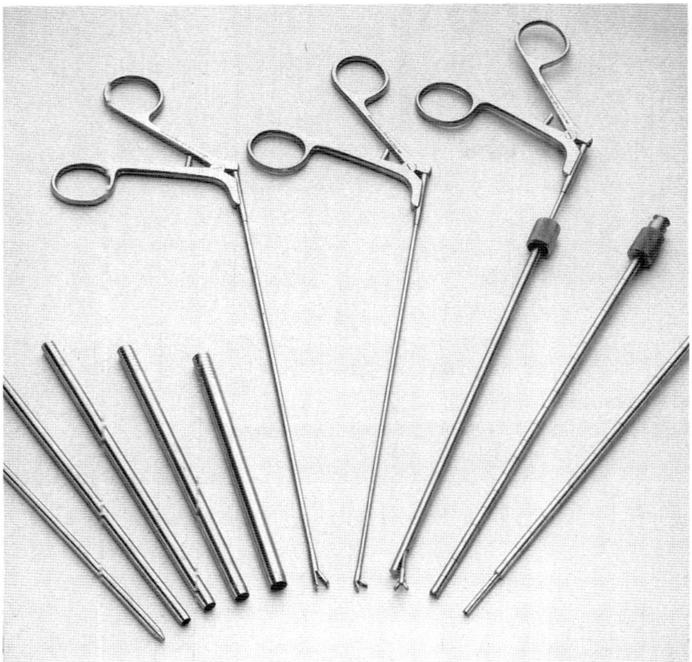

Fig. 2. Obturator with central drilling, working tubes of different diameters, straight and flexible forceps and annulus trephines (with permission of Aesculap Werke AG, Tuttlingen, FRG)

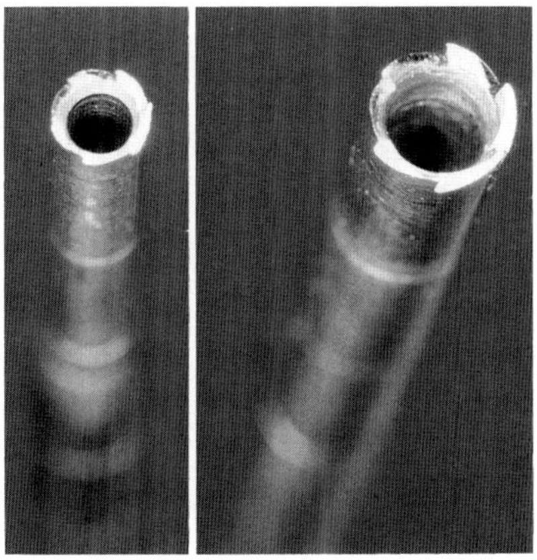

Fig. 3. Instrumentation for opening the intervertebral space

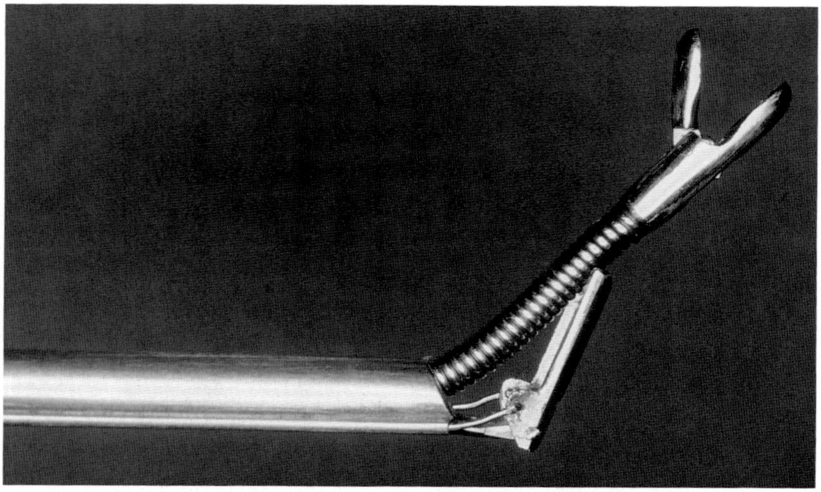

Fig. 4. Prototype of a flexible forceps with a wide-range deflector to reach the dorsal boundaries of the intervertebral space

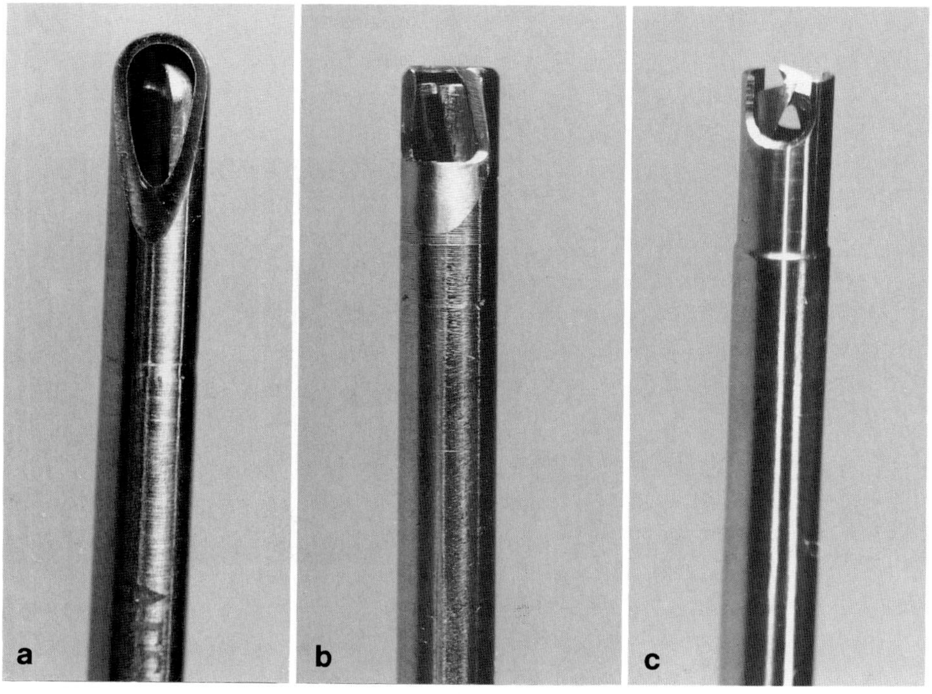

Fig. 5 a–c. Shavers of different shapes and sizes for the automated removal of nucleus pulposus

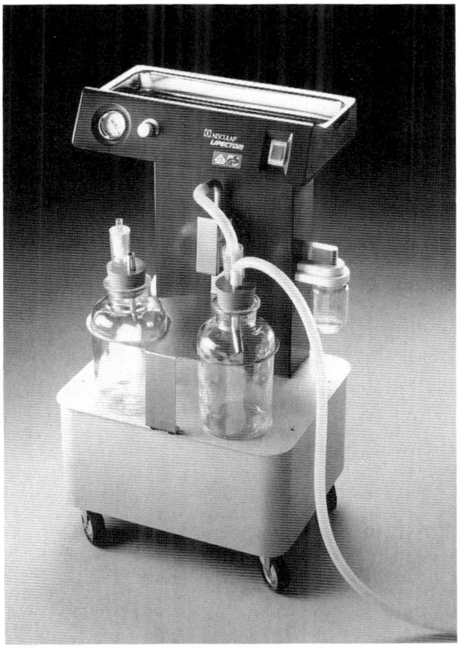

Fig. 6. High-powered surgical suction apparatus (Lipectom) which creates a 99% vacuum within 15 s (with kind permission of Aesculap Werke AG, Tuttlingen, FRG)

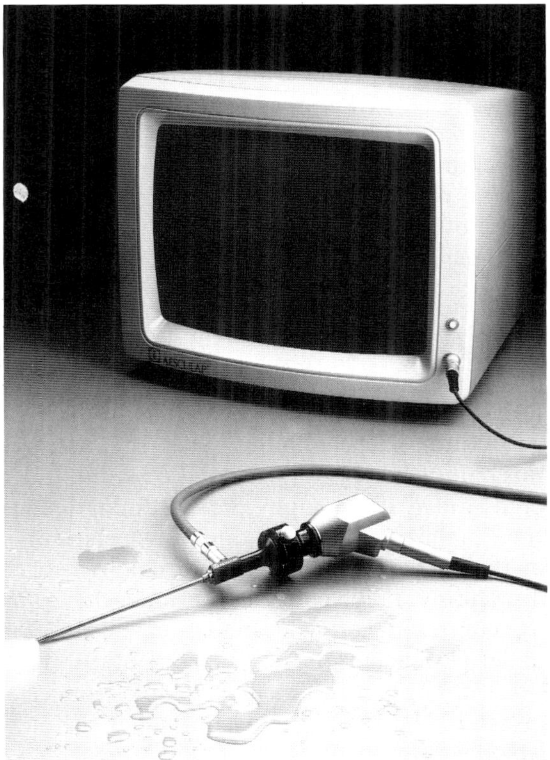

Fig. 7. CCD camera for videoscopic discoscopy (with kind permission of Aesculap Werke AG, Tu:tlingen, FRG)

Surgical Technique [8]

Patient Positioning

The patient is positioned in a comfortable prone position on a radiolucent operating table. Thorax and pelvis are propped with cushions in order to achieve flexion of the hip joints and compensate for lumbar lordosis. In paramedian herniations, the approach is always from the symptomatic side. In cases of medial disc herniations, the approach is from the side with the main symptoms. In intra- or extraforaminal herniations, the protruding nucleus pulposus may be localized in a "dead angle" for the ipsilateral posterolateral approach. In such cases, access from the opposite side might be advantageous. In patients with non-lateral symptoms, the approach usually is from the right side, where there is less danger of injury to retroperitoneal structures as compared to the left side (descending colon, sigmoid artery).

Posterolateral Approach

The projection on the skin of the level of the disc to be treated is marked under fluoroscopic control. The C-arm of the fluoroscope must be tilted to give a parallel projection of the vertebral end-plates, since the intervertebral space should be reached by the instruments parallel to the end-plates to avoid damage and erosion of these structures. The point of entrance is marked on the skin, 8 to 10 cm from the midline at the level of the intervertebral space. Skin and subcutaneous tissue are anesthesized with lidocaine (1%). *Although general anesthesia is contraindicated, an anesthesiologist must be on stand-by.* The intervertebral space is then punctured with the 18G cannula at an angle between 45° and 60° to the sagittal plane. The tip of the cannula must be located exactly in the geometric center of the disc. This is *the most important step of the operation,* since all further steps depend on the exact placement of the cannula.

Discography

Discography is routinely performed to exclude any possible perforation or sequestration in the epidural space. It is not necessary to perform discography at this point when perforation and/or sequestration have already been excluded by preoperative discography or post-discographic CT (disco-CT) (Fig. 8). Small fissures in the outer parts of annulus which result in a small, subligamentous deposit of the contrast medium do not comprise a contraindication for percutaneous discectomy. Large perforations under the ligament do, however, represent a relative contraindication [8]. In these cases, nucleectomy should at least be performed under permanent discoscopic control through a second percutaneous approach [14, 15]. The contrast medium should be injected carefully with slowly increasing pressure. One should inquire whether the patient experienced "memory pain", which we were able to provoke in about 50% of our cases.

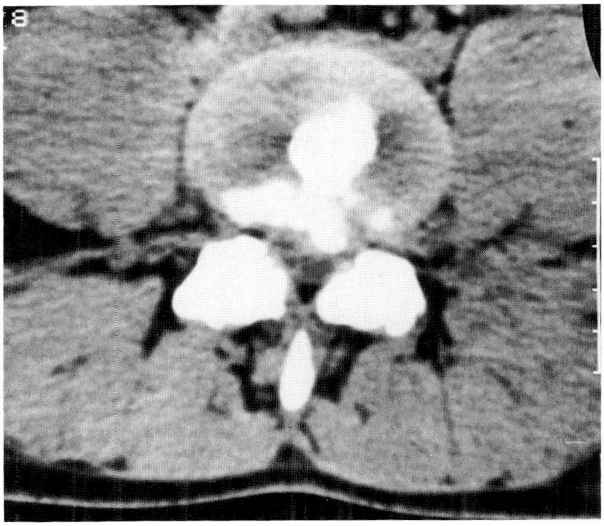

Fig. 8. Post-discographic CT (disco-CT) showing a protrusion through a wide degenerative cleft in the annulus fibrosus without signs of perforation into the epidural space

Insertion of Instruments

Following discography, the guide wire is introduced through the cannula, and the cannula is then removed. When removing the cannula, the guide wire must be held in place to prevent displacement. The point of entry of the wire is widened by a stab incision, so that the blunt obturator can be advanced down the disc using the wire as a guide. Again, the wire should be held in place with one hand to prevent it from traversing the intervertebral space. The tip of the obturator is advanced until the dorsolateral border of the disc is reached (Fig. 9). During this step, the surgeon may feel elastic resistance if the tip of the obturator presses against the annulus fibrosus, and the patient may experience pseudoradicular pain projecting into the buttock or the dorsal aspect of the thigh. *Caution: If there is radicular pain or sensory disturbance, the position of the obturator must be corrected in order to prevent injury to the nerve root.* The detachable Luer-lock adapter is removed from the obturator. The working tube is inserted using the obturator as a guide, then it is carefully advanced with rotating movements until its central opening can be gently pressed against the annulus fibrosus. The guide wire and the obturator are then removed while leaving the working cannula in place (Fig. 10).

Opening the Intervertebral Space

The annulus fibrosus is perforated with a small annulus trephine (OD 3 mm). If this is painful for the patient, a local anesthetic can be applied through the

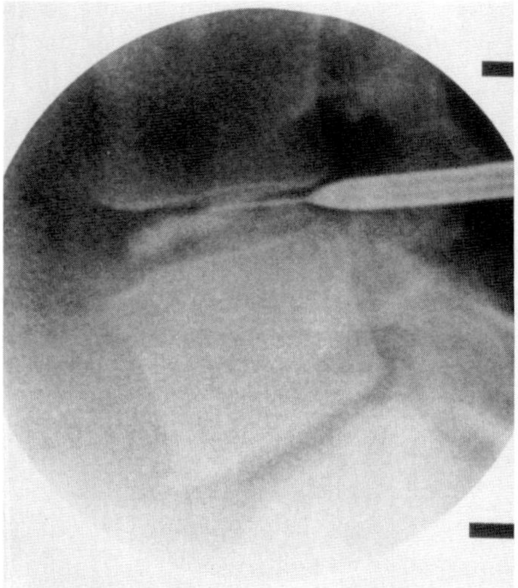

Fig. 9

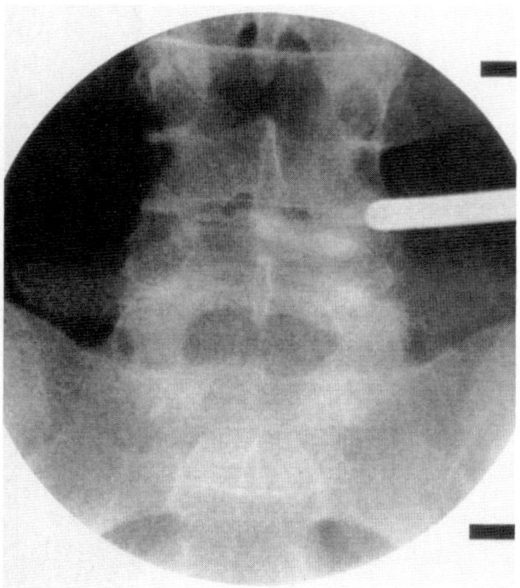

Fig. 10

Fig. 9. Guide wire and obturator in situ. The tip of the obturator is placed at the border of the disc L 4/L 5 in the lateral X-ray projection

Fig. 10. Working sleeve placed at L 4/L 5. A-P X-ray projection

trephine itself. The perforation is then enlarged, either with a large trephine (OD 4.5 mm) or with the automated trephine. A tissue cylinder can be obtained in most cases. Perforation of the annulus fibrosus and the protruding nucleus pulposus can be verified or disproved by discoscopy (Fig. 11).

Nucleectomy

The removal of nucleus pulposus is initiated with straight, or angled, rigid forceps and the shaver system (Fig. 12). A small cylindric cavity is thereby created in the center of the disc. Discoscopy can now be performed without difficulty, allowing the surgeon to check the amount of tissue remaining and spot any fragments in the dorsal area of the intervertebral space, which are then removed with flexible forceps. During discoscopy the patient is asked to press or cough, which, in most cases, evokes displacement of additional nucleus pulposus material from the dorsal parts towards the central intradiscal cavity, which can then be easily removed with the forceps or the shaver. The procedure is completed when no more material can be obtained by either manual or automated instruments. The working tube is then withdrawn and the stab incision is closed with a single suture.

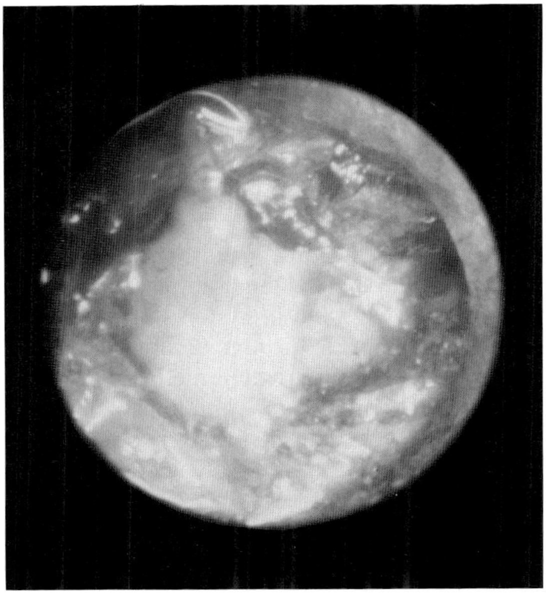

Fig. 11. Discoscopic view of a nucleus pulposus protruding through the perforated annulus fibrosus

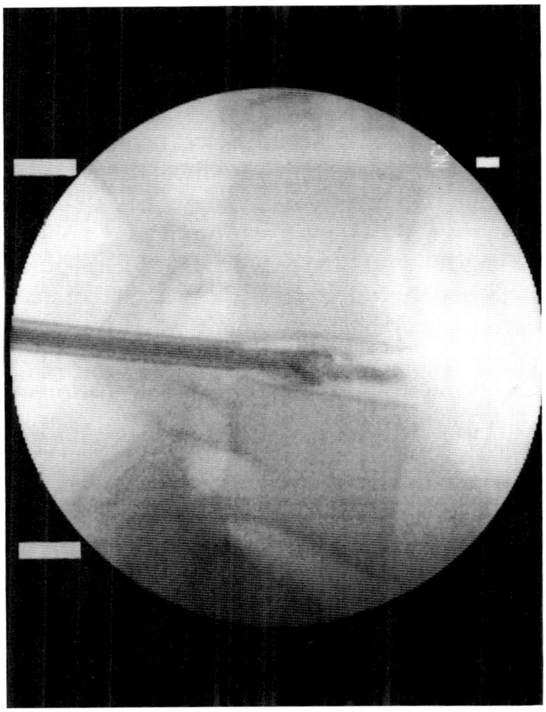

Fig. 12. Straight forceps in the center of the intervertebral space L4/L5. Lateral X-ray projection

Discussion

The percutaneous posterolateral approach to the lumbar intervertebral spaces opens a new dimension in the treatment of disc herniation. The technical challenges have led to different solutions comprising closed decompression of the intervertebral space or "open" percutaneous nucleectomy [5, 7, 13]. The introduction of a discoscope through a second contralateral approach extends the indication for PLD to prolapses perforated underneath the dorsal longitudinal ligament [14, 18]. The need for a technique which combines decompression, "open" and selective nucleectomy, the use of rigid and flexible instruments, the use of automated shaver and cutter systems, the application of high-powered suction and discoscopic control through a single approach arose from combining several advantages of the individual methods described hitherto.

The PLD methods of Kambin [5] or Hijikata [2] represent a partial nucleectomy with manual instruments (forceps). The procedure requires complete fluoroscopic control. Automated instruments are not used, discoscopic control is not performed. Schreiber and Suezawa [14, 17] introduced discoscopy to achieve visual control of the surgical procedure. However, the endoscope is introduced from the contralateral side and requires a second surgical approach, which prolongs the overall time of the procedure. Flexible instruments are not used routinely. Although a second approach to the disc space may be useful in intraforaminal disc protrusions or in cases of subligamentous perforation or sequestration, it does not seem to provide any advantages in routine PLD.

Automated percutaneous lumbar discectomy (APLD) represents another surgical variation [7, 13]. The disposable nucleotome probe can achieve "closed" decompression of the disc space. It is indicated in disc protrusion, and the efficacy can be compared to that of chemonucleolysis. It seems to be a safe procedure at the cost of limited indications. If used properly, only a central cylinder of nucleus pulposus will be removed. Since there is no permanent open decompression of the intervertebral space, an intradiscal rearrangement of the remaining nucleus material may cause a "self-sealing effect" [6]. Discoscopic control is not possible. Moreover, the intensity of the vacuum applied to the intervertebral space is not defined, and it is applied through a distal opening of only 2 mm in diameter. The L 5/S 1 space can be reached with a curved cannula, however, mere disc protrusions are fairly rare at the L 5/S 1 level (did not exceed 5% of the cases in our series).

Our surgical technique, using the instruments described, permits selective and controlled nucleectomy with a single approach. The amount of nucleus removed averaged 4–5 g [12]. X-ray exposure time decreased from 1.5 min in the first 30 patients to 60 s or less in the remainder. Between April 8, 1987 and December 31, 1988, a total of 64 patients were treated by percutaneous endoscopic lumbar discectomy (PELD). Except for one case of spondylodiscitis (which was successfully treated), no major complications were observed. Preliminary results observed after a minimum follow-up time of 6 months are promising [8–12]. The combination of this procedure with endoscopic laser technology opens new perspectives for atraumatic, safe and selective removal of even perforated lumbar disc herniations.

References

1. Friedman WA (1983) Percutaneous discectomy: an alternative to chemonucleolysis? Neurosurgery 13(5): 542–547
2. Hijikata SA (1975) A method of percutaneous nuclear extraction. J Toden Hosp 5: 39
3. Kambin P (1987) Mechanisms of pain relief and research aspect of annular fenestration and percutaneous discectomy. Int Symp on Percutaneous Discectomy. Philadelphia, USA, March 1987
4. Kambin P, Gellman H (1983) Percutaneous lateral discectomy of the lumbar spine. Clin Orth Rel Res 174: 127–132
5. Kambin P, Sampson S (1986) Posterolateral percutaneous suction excision of herniated intervertebral disc. Clin Orth Rel Res 207: 37–43
6. Markolf KL, Morris JM (1974) The structural components of the intervertebral disc. J Bone Joint Surg 56(A)4: 675–687
7. Maroon JC, Onik G (1987) Percutaneous automated discectomy: a new method for lumbar disc removal. J Neurosurg 66: 143–146
8. Mayer HM (1988) Perkutane Lumbale Diskektomie. Aesculap Werke AG, S 95, 12/88
9. Mayer HM (in press) Percutaneous lumbar discectomy in the treatment of discogenic low back pain and sciatica. In: Bartko T, Turcani P (eds) New Trends in Neurology. John Libbey & Co, London
10. Mayer HM, Brock M (1988) Behandlung des lumbalen Bandscheibenvorfalls – Die Perkutane Diskektomie. Deutsches Ärzteblatt 85(13): 853–858
11. Mayer HM, Brock M (1988) Percutaneous discectomy in the treatment of pediatric lumbar disc disease. Surg Neurol 29: 311–314
12. Mayer HM, Brock M (in press) Percutaneous endoscopic lumbar discectomy (PELD). In: Voth D et al. (eds) Neurosurgical Review. Walter de Gruyter, Berlin New York
13. Onik G, Helms CA, Ginsberg L, Hoaglund ET, Morris J (1985) Percutaneous lumbar discectomy using a new aspiration probe. AJNR 6: 290–293
14. Schreiber A, Suezawa Y (1986) Transdiscoscopic percutaneous nucleotomy in disc herniation. Orth Rev 15(1): 75–78
15. Schreiber A, Suezawa Y, Leu HJ (1988) Therapie des Bandscheibenprolaps – Chemonukleolyse versus perkutane Nukleotomie. DMW 113: 1482–1485
16. Shepperd JAN (1986) Posterolateral percutaneous surgery to the lumbar spine. Alternatives in Spinal Surgery 3: 4
17. Suezawa Y, Ruettimann B (1983) Indikation, Methodik und Ergebnisse der perkutanen Nukleotomie bei lumbaler Diskushernie. Z Orthop 126: 1–7
18. Suezawa Y, Schreiber A (1988) Perkutane Nukleotomie mit Diskoskopie. Z Orth 126: 1–7

Percutaneous Posterolateral Decompression for the Treatment of Chronic Low Back Pain of Discogenic Origin

A. MONTEIRO [1], G. PIETERS [2], and D. GASTAMBIDE [3]

Introduction

Amongst the large range of potential etiologies concerning chronic low back pain, with or without temporary sciatica, there is one cause that seldom comes in mind: the discogenic origin of the pain. Since 1978 we have maintained that the over-pressure inside the disc and the over-distension of the peridiscal ligamentous coats cause the local pain and are the source of the metameric painful reflexes. As a consequence, the logical treatment would be to decompress the disc by drilling a percutaneous lateral fenestration and a tunnel up to the nucleus for draining nuclear materials.

Materials and Methods

The role of the disc in the lumbar pain must be demonstrated clearly. After having eliminated the extra-vertebral causes and after having discussed the skeletal causes of lumbalgias, clinicians have to consider the possible involvement of the disc in the complaints.

Besides the standard X-rays whose reliability is poor for discopathy, the dynamic X-rays with bending test may demonstrate the flexibility or inflexibility of discs. Each disc is the center of the "functional unit" it makes with the two adjacent vertebrae and all their connecting ligaments. The suppleness of the unit depends on age and level considered. But only 40% of blocked discs are related to discopathy.

The rigid or blocked discs will undergo discography. This may show:

1. A normal disc.
2. A lateralized nucleus, a sign of a double nucleius (Fig. 1).
3. A degenerated asymptomatic nucleus (injection test negative).
4. A burst nucleus which can be a true intranuclear hernia under pressure, with a positive injection test.

[1] Rue de la Briqueterie 178, 6140 Fontaine-l'Evêque, Belgium
[2] Hôpital de Jumet, Service de Chirurgie Orthopédique, 6000 Charleroi, Belgium
[3] Hôpital de Blois, Service de Chirurgie Orthopédique, 41000 Blois, France

Percutaneous Lumbar Discectomy
Ed. by H. M. Mayer and M. Brock

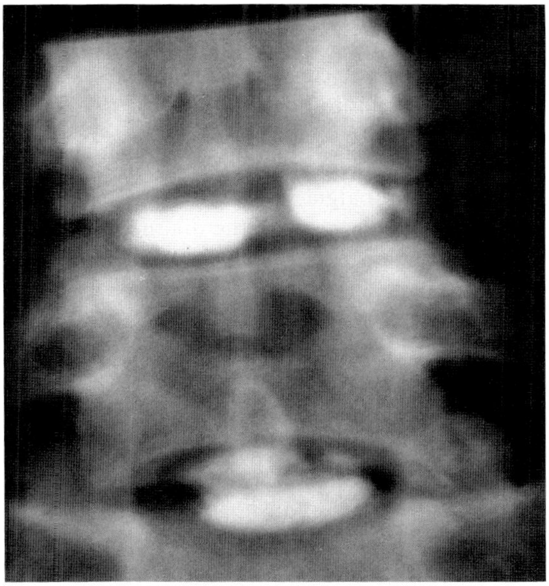

Fig. 1. Double nucleius

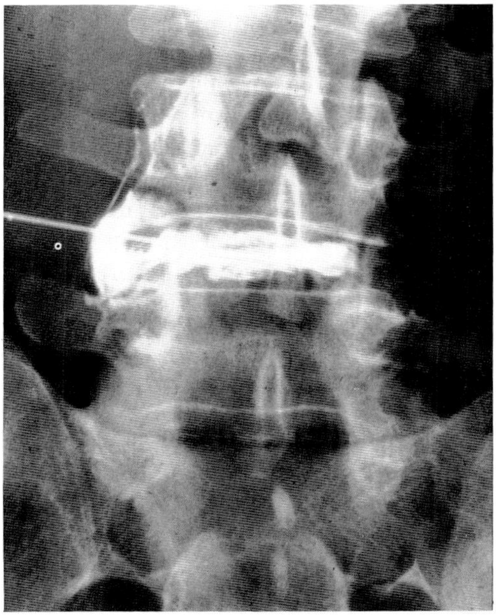

Fig. 2. Lateral hernia

5. A lateral or an anterior hernia (Fig. 2).
6. A postero-medial protrusion (without radicular syndrome) at one level. When at multiple levels, it sometimes generates a secondary narrow canal.
7. A posterolateral hernia as a cause of low back pain and sciatica.

Regarding the injection test, one knows that a healthy disc accepts no more than 0,5 to 1 ml of fluid (saline or contrast medium) and that the injection under slight pressure does not cause pain. In contrast a pathological nuclear chamber may take 2 or more ml and is painful.

The concordance of blocked disc, positive injection test (pain and amount injected) and image of pathological disc allows the affirmation of the discal origin of chronic lumbalgia.

Another way to reach the diagnosis is: low back pain, plus protrusion identified by CT scan, plus blocked disc, plus relief of pain when patient is in "suspension kyphosis" position. These four elements together give evidence of the discogenic origin of the complaints.

Technique

The technique of percutaneous posterolateral approach of lumbar discs was first described by S. Hijikata in 1975 [1]. We began applying it in 1978, operating first on lumbosciatical patients and later on pure chronic lumbalgias.

In contrast to some authors [2–4] we do not perform a total removal of the nucleus and we do not use a bilateral approach permitting a nucleoscopic control. We represent "the minimalist trend" of the technique. It means that after having reached the nucleus through a thin fenestration of the annulus, we only parcel the nucleus, letting bits of nuclear material escape spontaneously under axial pressure into the surrounding muscles where they can be phagocytized. This technique avoids best the risks of instability of the spine as well as the narrowing of the intervertebral space.

This technique of "simple nucleotomy", in contrast to the total nucleectomy, is a minimal invasive one. It lasts only 15 to 20 min, requires a hospital stay of 24 h and a very short period of recovery.

The following findings suggest that the abolition of the intra-discal over-pressure is the key to the cure:

1. Irrespective of the site of the pain, the result is the same whether the approach is ipsilateral or contralateral.
2. The result is not better with a symmetrical approach.
3. The amount of nuclear material withdrawn has no significance for the prognosis.

Clinical Data

Between 1978 and 1988 we operated on 210 patients complaining of simple, chronic, sometimes severe lumbalgias. The youngest was 20 years and the oldest 76 (average 43 years). There were 48% men and 52% women. They altogether had 339 pathological discs. Regarding the levels operated on during the same session, 97 patients were operated on at one level, 101 patients at 2 levels, 8 patients at 3 levels and 4 patients at 4 levels.

Medium and long-term results were very good in 73% of the cases and good in 23%.

Discussion

Lumbalgia is a globally perceived pain, a subjective reality that can generally be objectivized. It originates in a functional vertebral unit which is supple when sound and becomes a functional block when unbalanced, wherever the site of the original lesion. The site may be discal in 10% of the chronic cases. The lumbalgia without lesions clearly visualized by standard imaging techniques should induce a search for disc pathology. Likewise, it is conceivable that only a part of the declared pain is referred to the identified lesion.

Thus for instance, when low back pain persists after conventional surgery for lumbosciatalgia that resolved the sciatica problem, one should suspect that the remaining lumbalgia could be referred to a discopathy located at a level adjacent to the operated one.

Case Reports

1. Male, 49 years. Treated for two years for severe lumbalgia related to well identified (by standard X-ray) arthrosis (Fig. 3). Three positive tests indicating discopathy. Discotomy. Recovery (80%). Return to work.

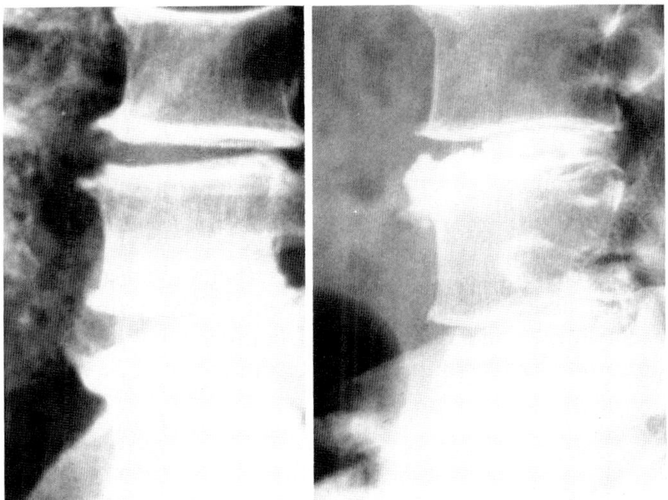

Fig. 3. Arthrosis, discopathy at L4–L5 and L5–S1 and anterior hernia at L4–L5

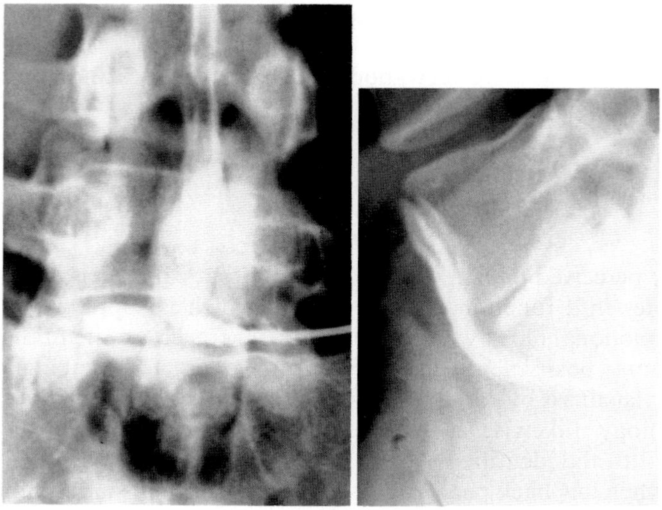

Fig. 4. Double nucleius with subligamentous suffusion from one of the nuclei

2. Female, 55 years. After 18 months suffering attributed to muscular rheumatism, submitted to the three tests, which were positive; image of double nucleus and anterior hernia from the right nucleus (Fig. 4). Discotomy. Recovery.
3. Male, 52 years. Operated on for slipped disc L 5–S 1. Persistence for more than 9 months of severe lumbalgia. Three tests positive for L 4–L 5. Discotomy. Recovery.
4. Male, 57 years. Severe lumbalgia: standard X-ray negative; bending test positive; discography negative. No indication for operation. Classical treatment for chronic rheumatism.

Conclusions

Chronic lumbalgias, moderate or severe, with or without easily identified lesions, may have a discal origin which is responsible partially or totally for the pain experienced.

Three successive positive tests (bending test, injection test and dislocated image) assert the disc involvement in the painful syndrome. The treatment according to the rationale and confirmed by the results consists in a simple discotomy for decompression. Results are good or very good in 96% of the cases.

References

1. Hijikata S, Yamagishi M, Nakayama T et al. (1975) Perkutane Nukleotomie – Neue Behandlung der Diskushernie. J Toden Hosp 5: 5–13
2. Kambin P, Gellman H (1983) Percutaneous lateral discectomy of the lumbar spine. A preliminary report. Clin Orth Rel Res 174: 127–132
3. Onik G, Maroon J, Helms C (1987) Automated percutaneous discectomy. Initial patient experience. Radiology 162: 129–132
4. Schreiber A, Suezawa Y (1986) Transdiscoscopic percutaneous nucleotomy in disc herniation. Orthop Rev 15: 35–38

Percutaneous Lumbar Discectomy and CT Discography

D. GASTAMBIDE [1], A. MONTEIRO [2], G. PIETERS [2], J.C. GARNIER [1], T. BENARDEAU [1], and R. MAILLARD [1]

The diagnosis of free hernia remains the most difficult problem in percutaneous lumbar surgery. We thought we could obtain better results by using systematic CT discography (CTD) before percutaneous lumbar discectomy [2–4].

We performed our first PLD in Blois in October 1987. To date, we have operated on 47 patients on 72 different levels using Monteiro's technique, which he first used in Charleroi (Hôpital de Jumet) on August 25th 1978.

Our first 10 patients did not undergo CTD. We obtained 6 good results, 3 fair, and 1 poor. We did not understand the reason for our poor result, and therefore began performing CTD systematically.

During the last five months, we performed CTD on 58 patients, each one undergoing at least 2 discograms.

Here, we report on the 52 cases operated on to date:

Three were accomplished before intersomatic percutaneous graft; 3 after PLD, with 1 good result, 1 fair, 1 poor. Both fair and poor results had no CTD before PLD.

We performed 46 CTD on candidates for PLD. Only 29 of these 46 candidates had a PLD (63%) because there were 8 contraindications and 9 undecided patients. The 8 contraindications to PLD consisted of 5 extruded hernias, 2 postsurgical fibrosis and 1 lumbar stenosis. Of the 9 undecided patients for PLD, 2 had been previously operated on for another hernia at another level, 4 preferred to wait one or two months for personal reasons, 2 noticed spontaneous improvement after CTD, and 1 had only intermittent symptomatology.

Of the 29 CTD followed by PLD, we nucleotomized 44 levels (15 patients had 2 nucleotomized levels), and 30 hernias were well opacified. The results were: 19 good, 8 fair, 2 poor.

Of these 29 patients, 5 presented isolated lumbalgia. We were surprised to see a great majority of well opacified hernias (9 nucleotomized levels) and obtained 5 good results. In these cases, the patients felt dramatically and definitively better in the hours after PLD.

The 24 other patients had lumbosciatalgias, with 22 improvements (14 good, 8 fair). There were 35 nucleotomized levels among 23 well opacified hernias. In the two failures, we noticed 2 poorly opacified hernias on the two nucleotomized levels.

[1] Hôpital de Blois, Service de Chirurgie Orthopédique, 41 000 Blois, France
[2] Hôpital de Jumet, Service de Chirurgie Orthopédique, 6000 Charleroi, Belgium

Percutaneous Lumbar Discectomy
Ed. by H.M. Mayer and M. Brock

The 5 free hernias seen on CTD showed no filling at disc level in 2 cases (1 with epidurography), poor filling in one case (less than 30%), and 2 migrated hernias.

Discussion

The CTD can determine whether the hernia communicates with the nucleus. When the hernia is well opacified, a good result can be expected.

When opacification is partial or poor, results are mediocre.

We hope to measure intradiscal pressure using Castagnera, Lavignolle, and Senegas's discomanometric technique in a few months [1].

Some Specific CTD Problems

Great pressure on the symptomatic disc with reproduction of the lumbalgia during discography, clinically suspected because of an increase in intervertebral height on standard X-rays, corresponding to a "balloonized disc" (Renier) [5]. We noticed such a case in a 36-year-old woman (Fig. 1).

The double nucleius. At first, we have to verify that there is no annulography, and then eliminate a lateralized nucleus associated with an intradiscal hernia (Fig. 2).

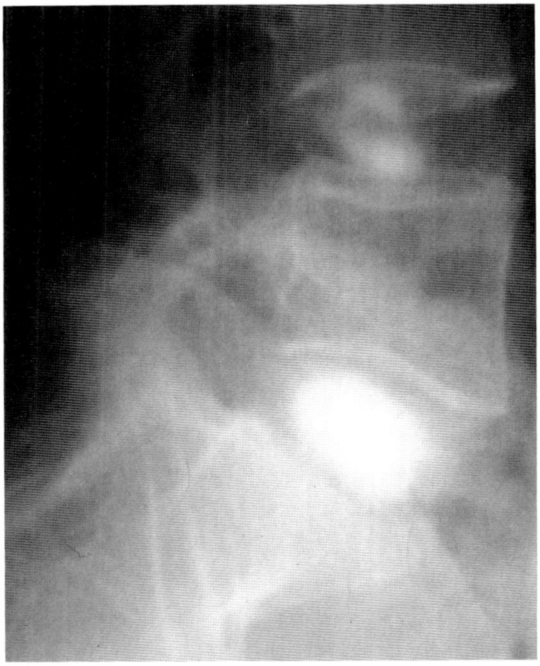

Fig. 1. "Balloonized disc" [5]. It was symptomatic during discography

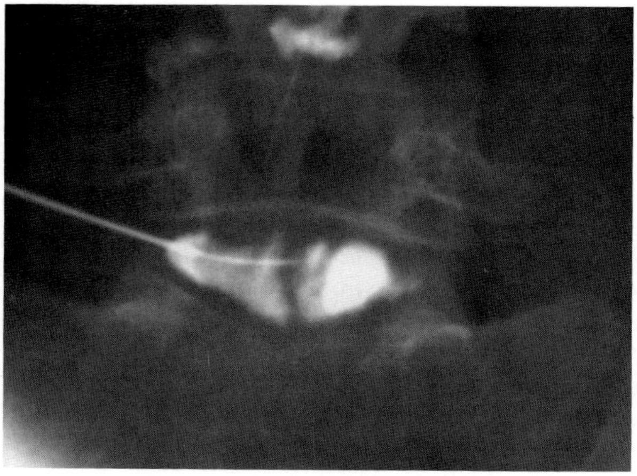

Fig. 2. "Double nucleius" or lateralized nucleus with intradiscal hernia on the other side?

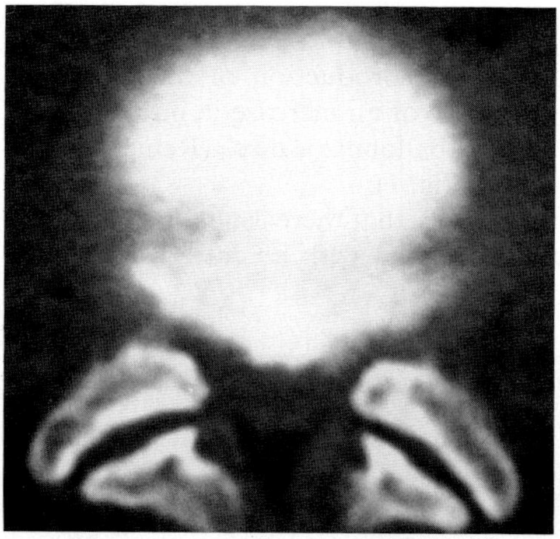

Fig. 3. CTD before PLD

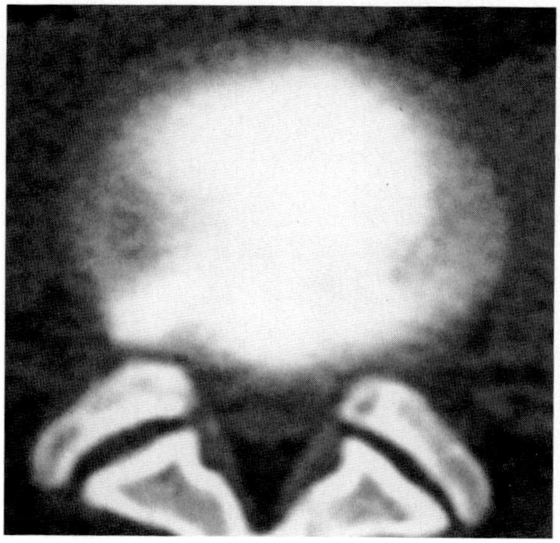

Fig. 4. CTD two months after PLD

CTD is indicated in cases of predominantly radicular pain following a standard X-ray, and a CT scan to show the level. CTD may show that there is no extruded hernia.

In predominant lumbalgias, we perform a standard X-ray centered on each pathological disc. The asymmetry of one or two discs shows the level to study with CTD.

If discography is symptomatic and the hernia well opacified, a good result can be expected. The CTD can show something other than a posterior hernia, for example, a lateral or anterior hernia which can be associated with abdominal pain or groin pain.

Finally, one patient had CTD before and after PLD. This resulted in decreased intervertebral disc height (less than 20%), a decreased hernia at the L4–L5 level, and a picture of the PLD trajectory (Figs. 3, 4).

Conclusions

Of course, CTD and PLD should be proposed only after failure following two or three months of medical treatment.

CTD is essential in isolated lumbalgia when pain recurs during discography. When the hernia is well opacified, we can be sure that we will have an immediate and lasting good result.

In the lumboradiculalgias, the best results are in well opacified hernias. Incomplete or poorly opacified filling has no predictive value. If there is no filling at all, the hernia is excluded.

In the future workshops of the European "Percutaneous Nucleotomy" association, we hope to standardize the patient examination form.

References

1. Castagnera L, Lavignolle B, Vital JM, Grenier F, Baulny D, Senegas J (1988) Etude fonctionnelle du disque pathologique par la discomanométrie. Revue du Rhumatisme 55(5): 981–988
2. Colhoun E, McCall IW, Williams L, Cassar Pullicino VN (1988) Provocation discography as a guide to plan operations of the spine. J bone joint surg 70-B(2): 267–271
3. Edwards WC, Prame TJ, Orr Edwards G (1987) CT discography: prognostic value in the selection of patients for chemonucleolysis. Spine 12: 792–795
4. Michael E, McCutcheon, Thompson WC (III) (1986) CT scanning of lumbar discography, a useful diagnostic adjunct. Spine 11(3): 257–258
5. Renier JC, Audran M, Dajon JL, Bureau Th (1988) Le disque ballonné. Une étiologie du tableau de l'homme raide. Revue du rhumatisme 55(8): 585–588

Differential Indication for Chemonucleolysis and Percutaneous Discotomy According to the Behavior of the Nucleus After Treatment

A. Hedtmann [1], H.-J. Fischer [2], and J. Krämer [1]

Summary

Out of 100 patients of a randomized, prospective study of collagenase (CO) and chymopapain (CH) in the intradiscal treatment of symptomatic lumbar disc disease, 51 were followed up for two years by repetitive MRI studies (16 patients after collagenase and 35 after chymopapain). These were compared with a preliminary three months follow-up of 6 patients after percutaneous discotomy (PD). The reduction of size of herniation during the first month/after three months was about 50%/– (CO), 55%/70% (CH), and 9%/22% (PD). The reduction of nucleus size after one month/three months was about 19%/– (CO), 42%/66% (CH) and 18%/15% (PD).

The height of IVS was reduced after one month/three months for about 21%/– (CO), 18%/33% (CH), and 0%/8% (PD).

Conclusion: The efficacy of percutaneous discotomy regarding reduction of nucleus size, size of herniation and height of IVS is less than that of either chymopapain and collagenase. Patients with radicular symptoms associated with secondary signs of lumbar disc degeneration due to anatomical disintegration of disc structure like facet pain and instability symptoms might benefit more from percutaneous discotomy.

Introduction

During 1985/1986, a randomized comparative study of intradiscal therapy with either collagenase (CO; 400 ABC units) or chymopapain (CH 4000 IU) for symptomatic lumbar disc prolapse was conducted [2, 3]. 51 patients were followed up by repetitive investigations for about 2 years by magnetic resonance imaging (MRI) studies [1]. Seven patients who underwent percutaneous lumbar discotomy (PD) on the Level L 4/L 5 during the first half of 1988 were followed up by MRI repetitively for about 3 months.

The average age of patients was 34 years (CO), 29 years (CH) and 33 years (PD).

[1] Orthopädische Universitätsklinik Bochum, St. Josef-Hospital, Gudrunstraße 56, 4630 Bochum, FRG

[2] Institut für Kernspintomografie, Medizinische Fakultät, Universität Witten/Herdecke, 5804 Herdecke, FRG

Percutaneous Lumbar Discectomy
Ed. by H.M. Mayer and M. Brock

Methods

All MRI studies after chemonucleolysis cases were done on a device with a 0.5-tesla superconductive magnet with a body coil and a field of view of 30 cm. The studies after percutaneous discotomy were done either by the same device or alternatively on a 1.5-tesla superconductive machine. For intraindividual comparison, only series with the same imaging device were used. Imaging was done in the spin echo mode (T 1 and T 2 weighted) and in axial and sagittal projections. The size of the nucleus was determined as maximum extension in the T 2 images in sagittal projections. The size of herniation was measured in T 2 images as maximum extension in sagittal projection. In chemonucleolysis cases, the relative water content of the nucleus was measured additionally as spin density (rho), and the results are published elsewhere [1]. Calculations of water content after percutaneous discotomy are still under evaluation and will be published later.

Including criteria for chemonucleolysis (CN) and percutaneous discotomy were: clear signs of radicular pain arising from one of the three lower lumbar levels (CN)/arising from L 4/L 5 level (PD); no progressive or severe motor deficits; corresponding finding of lumbar discogenic root compression in the CT or MRI scan; at least six weeks of adequate conservative orthopedic treatment. Excluding criteria were: signs of free sequestration in the CT or MRI; pregnancy; spinal stenosis; severe neurologic deficit; advanced bony reactions of disc degeneration; previous open lumbar disc surgery.

Chemonucleolysis and percutaneous discotomy both were done under common operative conditions (operating room, draping) and general anesthesia after previous discography to assure proper intradiscal needle placement and to exclude free sequestrations. Fluoroscopy was done in two planes.

Percutaneous discotomy was done with mechanical instruments and powered sets for shaving with intermittent suction. No concomitant discoscopy was performed.

Postoperative ambulation was allowed from the first day. Aftercare comprised physical exercises (isometric trunk muscle training), back school, and bracing with an delordosing active orthosis (Lumboflex) for three months.

Results

One of the 7 cases followed up by repetitive MRI after PD had to be excluded from this series because he developed clinical signs of discitis, which could be confirmed by conventional x-rays as well as by MRI. Diagnostic disc puncture revealed no bacterial organisms. The patient recovered slowly over a period of 4 months but still is suffering from radicular symptoms which can easily be explained by the persisting disc protrusion.

Chymopapain leads to the greatest reduction of nucleus size, followed by collagenase. In the remaining 6 cases of percutaneous discotomy the comparatively lowest reduction of nucleus material (Fig. 1) was achieved. These relations

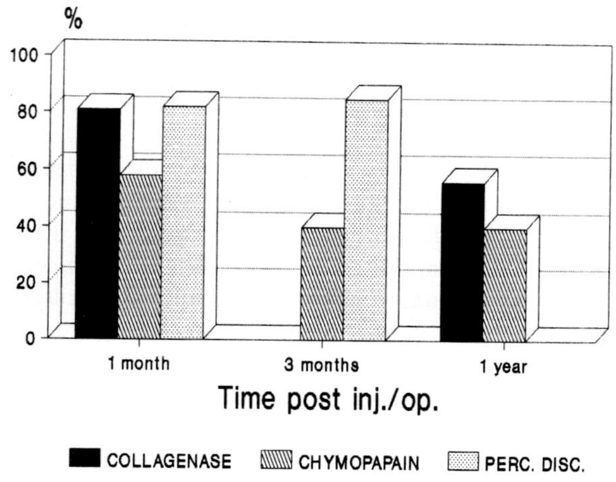

Fig. 1. Reduction of nucleus size after chemonucleolysis and percutaneous discotomy

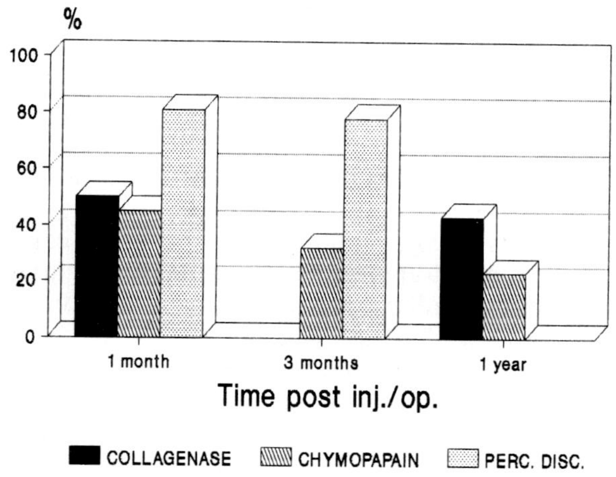

Fig. 2. Reduction of size of discal herniation after chemonucleolysis and percutaneous discotomy

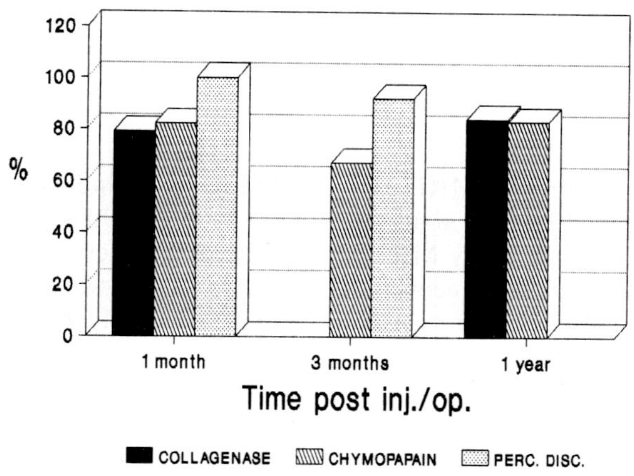

Fig. 3. Reduction of height of intervertebral space after chemonucleolysis and percutaneous discotomy

seemed to be unchanged for the first three months. In comparison to chymopapain, the process of reduction of nucleus size after percutaneous discotomy seems to be finished during the first month After three months, there seems to be no further reduction. In contrast, the reduction of nucleus size after chemonucleolysis with collagenase continues for about one year (Fig. 1).

The same is true for the size of herniation after chemonucleolysis, which decreases during the whole first year after treatment (Fig. 2) with either substance. The effect of percutaneous discotomy concerning reduction of hernial size is delayed in comparison to reduction of nuclear size as it can be observed in chemonucleolysis, but is much less than with the nucleus dissolving agents.

The reduction of intervertebral space (IVS) (Fig. 3) after chemonucleolysis is clearly dependent on the reduction of nuclear size, as previously described [1, 4].

Discussion

Regarding the reduction of nuclear size, disc herniation, and height of IVS, chemonucleolysis seems to be superior to percutaneous discotomy. This, probably, is the result of the present imperfect technical performance of PD: for anatomical reasons, percutaneous discotomy via the posterolateral approach reaches only the anterior half of the disc space. This is of special importance because herniation leads to a dislocation of the parts of the nucleus in posterior direction, so that a greater amount of disc material can be found in the posterior half of the nucleus. The chemonucleolytic agents, in contrast, have the ability to penetrate even to the posterior subligamentous structures, which enables efficacy even in the presence of subligamentous sequestrations of disc material which generally leads to poor results after PD [5].

Percutaneous discotomy obviously causes only a slight, almost negligible reduction of the height of intervertebral disc space. The limited number of investigated cases and the preliminary nature of the available data after percutaneous discotomy seem to support the hypothesis that the same mechanism of dependency of intervertebral space on nuclear size as seen in chemonucleolysis is true after PD, too.

Hypothetically, the lower reduction of nucleus volume after PD may be of specific value concerning some of the well-known side effects of chemonucleolysis such as increased or prolonged back pain, newly affected facet pain, which can be observed transiently in about 20% of cases after chemonucleolysis [3]: The lower reduction of disc height diminishes the increased facet load, which can be observed after either disc material removing procedure. The lower reduction of nuclear material may limit the therapeutic effect of root decompression, but preserves a greater amount of pre-tension of the annulus fibers, thus reducing the risk of postoperative instability syndromes. The lower reduction of intervertebral space after PD makes it a suitable procedure even in cases with a relatively narrowed lateral recessus, which is a common reason of therapeutic failure after chemonucleolysis, due to decompensation of the stenotic spinal canal in spite of adequate reduction of protruded disc material. The differential indications for chemonucleolysis and percutaneous discotomy on the basis of these preliminary data are:

Chemonucleolysis
- Large volume of herniation
- Subligamentous sequestration

Percutaneous discotomy
- Contained protrusions
- Radicular pain associated with
  - facet syndrome
  - instability
- Discogenic root compression associated with relative spinal stenosis.

References

1. Fischer HJ, Hedtmann A, Steffen R, Busch M, Scherer M (1987) Magnetic resonance imaging after chemonucleolysis and discolysis. Paper, presented to the 73rd Scient. Assemb. of the Radiol. Society of North America, Chicago, 1987
2. Hedtmann A, Steffen R, Krämer J (1982) Prospective comparative study of intradiscal high-dose and low-dose collagenase versus chymopapain. Spine 12: 388–392
3. Hedtmann A, Schleberger R, Wilcke A (1986) Nachbehandlung und Rehabilitation nach lumbaler Chemonukleolyse, in: Schleberger R, Krämer J (eds) Chemonukleolyse. Enke, Stuttgart, pp 95–113
4. Hedtmann A, Fischer HJ, Steffen R, Krämer J (1988) Magnetic resonance imaging after chemonucleolysis with chymopapain and collagenase. Paper presented to the XV. Ann. Meet. of the Int Soc for the Study of the Lumbar Spine (ISSLS), Miami 1988
5. Wiltse LL (1988) Results of chemonucleolysis in the USA and Canada. Paper, presented to the Int Symp on "5 years of Chemonucleolysis in Germany", 38. Jahrestagung der Vereinigung Nordwestdeutscher Orthopäden, Bochum, 1988

Results of Percutaneous Lumbar Discectomy Compared to Laminotomy and Chemonucleolysis

M. Swiecicki [1]

Introduction

The data for this analysis have been accumulated for a critical evaluation of the results of surgery that has been performed for lumbar disc herniation over the past five years. The patients included in this study each had one of four techniques employed. The techniques have included percutaneous lumbar discectomy, automated percutaneous lumbar discectomy, lumbar laminotomy or chemonucleolysis.

The data have been collected from patient records and patient follow-up surveys. They particularly focus on the length of conservative therapy prior to surgical intervention, and the length of hospital stay after surgery, and the percentage of patients in each group that have been able to return to work or resume their normal activities if they were never officially employed prior to the onset of their symptomatology. The average length of the recovery period has also been included in the evaluation for those patients who returned to work.

Materials and Methods

The data base for this evaluation includes one hundred consecutive patients in each group making a total of three hundred patients surveyed. The percutaneous lumbar discectomy group is subdivided into eighty-five automated procedures and fifteen nonautomated procedures for a total of one hundred percutaneous procedures.

The procedures performed upon these patients were all performed by the same surgeon in the same urban hospital complex. The information has been accumulated by my staff and has been entered into an IBM-PC computer utilizing a Professional File System. It was then subsequently evaluated by a data analyst.

The procedures have all been performed on patients with documented disc pathology by clinical evaluation as well as radiological evaluations. In each case at least two positive radiologic studies were obtained for confirmation of the findings. These studies included CT scanning, myelography, CT myelography,

[1] Hahnemann University, Department of Neurological Surgery, Philadelphia, PA 19102-1192, USA

Percutaneous Lumbar Discectomy
Ed. by H. M. Mayer and M. Brock

and MRI scanning. In most instances the patient's evaluation also included electromyography.

The patient selection strictly followed the guidelines proposed in the Postgraduate Course on Intradiscal Therapy which was sponsored as a joint effort by the American Assocation of Neurological Surgeons and American Academy of Orthopedic Surgeons and published in Chicago in 1982 [5].

Techniques

Automated percutaneous lumbar discectomies were performed in the operating room utilizing the Nucleotome System [2] and accessories with the technique described by Maroon [4, 6]. The percutaneous lumbar discectomies were performed with a Kambin Spinal Instrument Set [3], utilizing the Kambin [1–3] technique.

Disposable intradiscal needles were utilized for the chemonucleolysis with the occasional employment of the double needle technique. The procedures were all performed with Chymopapain [4]. Standard technique and instrumentation were employed for the conventional procedures. Magnification techniques were accomplished with a Wild or Zeiss microscope or surgical loupes.

The C-arm of the fluoroscope and image intensifier were utilized in all cases including the standard procedures. The percutaneous lumbar discectomies were performed with local anesthesia and supplemental intravenous techniques. The chemonucleolysis and lumbar laminotomies were performed under general endotracheal anesthesia.

Results

The patient population for this series had an average age of forty-three years, and each individual subgroup had an average age in the mid-forties. There was a nearly equal division in each of the groups of these procedures between male and female patients. More than half of the procedures involved the L4–5 disc and approximately one-third involved the L5–S1 disc.

Conservative therapy prior to surgical intervention in this group of patients with herniated lumbar discs was surprisingly protracted over an average length of 10.6 months. It was however uniform in each of the subgroups that were studied.

There was an average duration of pre-operative unemployment prior to any surgical intervention of 5.8 months with the shortest average time being

---

[2] Nucleotome Probe manufactured by Surgical Dynamics, San Leandro, California, USA

[3] Kambin Spinal Instrument Set manufactured by Pilling, Philadelphia, Pennsylvania, USA

[4] Chymopapain (Chymodiactin) produced by Smith Laboratories, Inc., Northbrook, Illinois, USA

3.4 months for those patients undergoing automated percutaneous lumbar discectomy.

The average length of hospital stay was counted from the day of surgery and included the day of discharge. The average for the entire series was five days of hospitalization. The automated percutaneous lumbar discectomies required the shortest period of hospitalization, with the average being two days. These patients were admitted on the day of surgery and discharged the following morning. The longest length of stay was the group that underwent lumbar laminotomy and the average for this group was seven days.

78.25% of the entire group of the three hundred patients returned to work. The highest category for returning to work was the group that had automated percutaneous lumbar discectomy, 83.5% of the patients in this group returned to work. The patients that had chemonucleolysis had the lowest percentage of return to work, averaging 58%, 75% of the laminotomy patients returned to work, a percentage just below the overall average.

The average length of unemployment post-operatively was 2.3 months. The recuperation averaged three months for laminotomy and 1.1 month for automated percutaneous lumbar discectomy making the recovery from automated percutaneous lumbar discectomy almost two months shorter than that for laminotomy and one and one half months shorter than chemonucleolysis.

During the recuperation period post-operatively, 32% of the overall patient population required physical therapy. 37% of the chemonucleolysis and laminotomy groups required physical therapy post-operatively, while only 15.3% of the automated percutaneous lumbar discectomy group required physical therapy.

The overall results of the surgical procedures as evaluated in this study are summarized in Figs. 1 and 2.

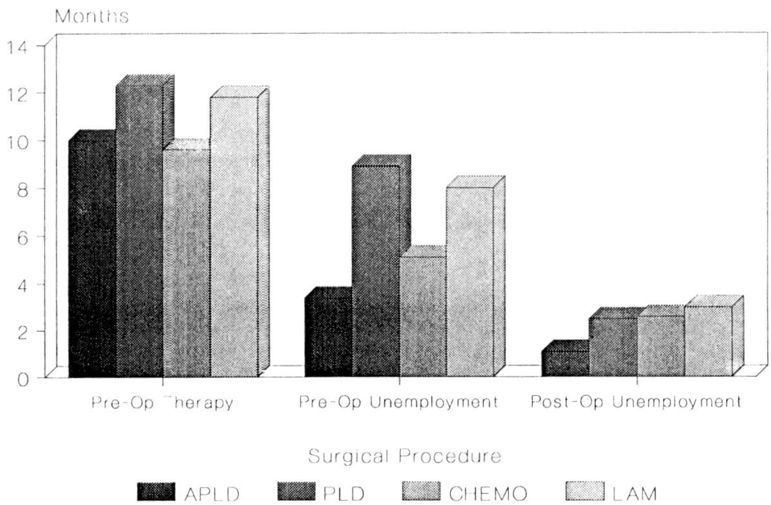

Fig. 1. Months of pre- and post-op care

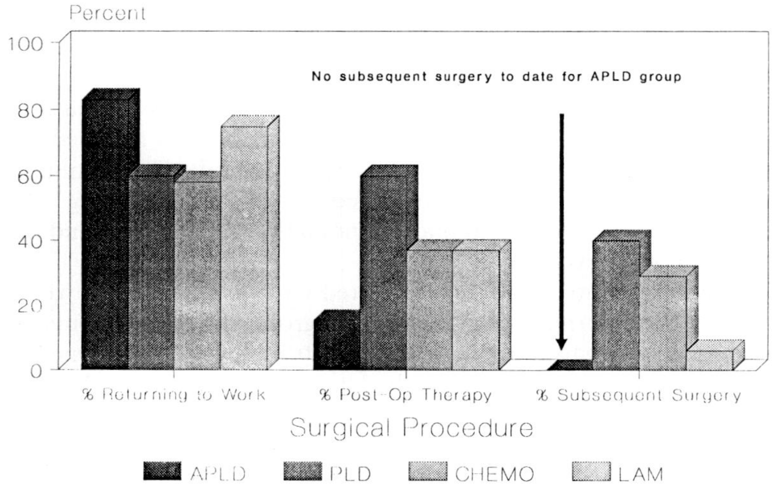

Fig. 2. Comparative data

Discussion

A comparison of the results of the techniques for the treatment of herniated lumbar disc has been performed to assess the value of the percutaneous methods in comparison to a standard type of open surgical procedure and method of dissolution of the disc.

The conclusions of this examiner drawn from this evaluation are based on the clinical status of the patients post-operatively and their ability to return to gainful employment or their normal activities in the shortest period of time. Although there were patients that were improved by each of the procedures, the highest percentage of patients improved were in the group that underwent automated percutaneous lumbar discectomy. This group of patients also averaged the shortest hospitalization and the shortest recovery period before returning to work.

The group that underwent chemonucleolysis had a longer recovery period than those that underwent an automated percutaneous lumbar discectomy although it was also shorter than the recovery period from laminotomy. The chemonucleolysis group however had the lowest percentage of patients returning to work.

At the time of this writing none of the patients that have undergone automated percutaneous lumbar discectomy have had a significant complication and none of them have had a repeat surgical procedure performed, although the follow-up on these patients has not been as long as it has been for any other category.

In summary, the data reflects the efficacy of the percutaneous approach as reflected in the short term follow-up on the patients that were operated on in this series. The procedure gives every indication of being an effective way of treating herniated lumbar discs and it is anticipated that the patients included in this series will be the subject of a long term follow-up.

The percutaneous method of disc removal compares very favorably with laminotomy for the treatment of lumbar disc herniation. It has required a much shorter recovery period and has enabled patients to return to work more rapidly. The shorter hospitalization and recovery period is beneficial to the patient and the treating physicians.

Acknowledgements. Acknowledgement to James A. Whelpley, BS, MBA, Systems Analyst; Diane M. Harris, BA, RN and Neurosurgical Associates Staff for the preparation of this paper.

This study is dedicated to Norman Eckbold, M.D., former Chief of Orthopedics Service, West Jersey Health System for his encouragement and support.

References

1. Friedman WA (1983) Percutaneous discectomy – an alternative to chemonucleolysis. J Neurosurgery 13: 542–547
2. Joson RA (1987) Percutaneous lumbar discectomy. Personal communication
3. Kambin P, Sampson S (1986) Posterolateral percutaneous suction – excision of herniated lumbar intervertebral discs. Clinical Orthopedics 207: 37–42
4. Maroon JC, Onik G (1987) Percutaneous automated discectomy: a new method for lumbar disc removal. J Neurosurgery 56: 143–146
5. Nordby EA (1982) Post-graduate course on intradiscal therapy, Chicago
6. Onik G, Maroon J, Helm C et al. (1987) Automated percutaneous discectomy: initial patient experience. Radiology 162: 129–132

Correlations of the Amount of Disc Removed by Percutaneous Lumbar Discectomy and Clinical Results

A. H. Capanna and D. M. Capanna [1]

Abstract

The amount of disc removed at percutaneous discectomy did not seem to correlate with the end clinical results of patients. A randomized, prospective analysis of patients end clinical results correlated with the amount of disc removed was undertaken. Disc material was all analyzed based on weight in grams.

All patients were evaluated by the authors. A comparative analysis between ten percutaneous discectomies and ten microdiscectomies was conducted. Similar results were obtained with either technique but a greatly reduced morbidity, cost, and a more rapid return to work were obtained with percutaneous discectomy.

Methods and Materials

A randomized prospective analysis of the ten percutaneous lumbar discectomies and ten microdiscectomies was carried out. All patients in succession were analyzed, and if surgery was performed, none could be eliminated from the study for any reason. Age, sex, level of disc removal, grams of disc removed, and results were all correlated. Results were termed: Excellent (no complaints); Good (normal function with minor, occasional compliants); Fair (some improvement, but continued complaints); Poor (no improvement or worse). Evaluation of return to work date postsurgically was carried out.

Percutaneous discectomies were all done as outpatients, with local anesthesia. The suction-aspiration technique and probe developed by Onik [7] was utilized. The microdiscectomies were performed by the technique developed by Williams [8] and Capanna [1–3]. All were done as inpatients with discharge from hospital one to three days postoperatively.

[1] The University of Nevada School of Medicine, Division Neurosurgery, 2040 W. Charleston Blvd., Suite 403, Las Vegas, NV 89102, USA

Percutaneous Lumbar Discectomy
Ed. by H. M. Mayer and M. Brock

Results

Microdiscectomies

The age range was 24 to 66 years (mean = 40) with a male to female ratio of three to seven. The levels of disc removal were: five at L 5–S 1, two at L 4–L 5, and three at L 4–5 and L 5–S 1. The grams of disc materal removed ranged from 3–20 grams (average = 8.15).

The clinical results were six excellent and four good, with no fair or poor results. The least amount of disc removed (3 g) was in a 50 year old male who had an excellent result. The largest amount of disc material removed (20 g) was in a 34 year old female with good results. There was no correlation with the amount of disc removed and clinical results.

The return to work was evaluated in seven of the ten patients (who had jobs). Of these, the range was 44 to 92 days, with an average of 65.4 days.

Percutaneous Discectomies

The age range was 26 to 56 years (mean = 37.5), with a male to female ratio of four to six. The levels of disc removal were: one at L 5–S 1, eight at L 4–L 5, and one at L 3–L 4. The amount of disc material removed ranged from less than 1 g to 18 g (average = 6.0 g).

The clinical results were five excellent, three good, two fair and no poor results. The least amount of disc removed was less than 1 g in three cases (2 excellent, one fair). The largest amount of disc removed (18 g) had only a good result. There was no correlation with the amount of disc removed and clinical results.

The return to work was evaluated in all ten cases. The range was 1 to 42 days, with an average of 18.8 days.

One of the fair results was in a physician who had 13 g of disc material removed. Postoperatively he had no back pain with some radicular pain completely relieved with steroids. The persistent (though decreased) radicular pain prompted a magnetic resonance scan which revealed a free fragment of disc. At microdiscectomy the fragment was removed and an empty disc space was noted. The patient then had an excellent result and now is a devout opponent of the percutaneous procedure!

Conclusions

A prospective analysis of this limited number of patients does not allow for specific conclusions which must await for greater number of patients. However, some generalizations can be deduced. The pércutaneous discectomy group was younger (average 2.5 years) possible secondary to less confusion about bony changes during there work-up. The average amount of disc removed showed little difference between percutaneous discectomy (6.0 g) versus microdiscectomy (8.15 g).

The clinical results between the two groups showed little difference. The major advantages of the percutaneous procedure over the microdiscectomy procedure were: 1) it was done as outpatient surgery, greatly reducing morbidity and costs, and 2) the return to work was 46.6 days shorter (or 3.5 times faster). The other advantage of percutaneous discectomy would appear to be a decreased, or possibly eliminated chance of future scarring of the nerve or neural canal.

It appears clear that the results of percutaneous discectomy should eliminate the use of chemonucleolysis [4]. The initial work with percutaneous discectomy [5, 6] seems to have been justified. The biggest problem will be in patient selection, particularly with the need to identify patients with free fragments of disc material.

References

1. Capanna AH (1980) Microlumbar discectomy in rats. J Microsurg 1: 351–353
2. Capanna AH (1984) Microlumbar discectomy. In: Olszewski W (Ed) Handbook of Microsurgery. CRC Press, Boca Raton/FL, pp 259–262
3. Capanna AH, Williams RW, Austin DC, Darmody WR, Thomas LM (1981) Radiographic calculation of the percentage of disc removal during lumbar discectomy and detection of anterior annulus perforation. Spine 6: 6
4. Friedman WA (1983) Percutaneous discectomy: an alternative to chemonucleolysis? Neurosurgery 13/5: 542–547
5. Hijikata SA (1975) A method of percutaneous nuclear extraction. J Toden Hospital 5: 39
6. Kambin P, Gellman H (1983) Percutaneous lateral discectomy of the lumbar spine. Clin Orth Rel Res 174: 127–132
7. Onik G, Helms CA, Ginsberg L, Hoaglund I, Morris J (1985) Percutaneous lumbar discectomy using a new aspiration probe. Am J Radiol 144: 1137–1142
8. Williams RW (1978) Microlumbar discectomy. A conservative surgical approach to the virgin herniated lumbar disc. Spine 3/2: 175

Differential Indication for Percutaneous Lumbar Discectomy

M. WEIGERT [1]

The importance of being earnest in performing new methods of treating disc disease can be seen in sensational reports of newspapers and television and in hostile reactions of disappointed patients. Especially in such a large city as Berlin, where specialists for the spine are to be found in at least ten clinics, a bad result immediately forces the patient to go from one hospital to another and not seldom the danger arises for a modern method, and also the physician, to be discriminated. In order to avoid such risks as far as possible, we handle every new procedure extremely cautiously with restrictive deliberations.

Five years ago, we began to practice chemonucleolysis according to the rules of the German Orthopedic Association. Excluding hyperergic reactions by prick and RAST test and routine discography, we treated 142 patients, 28 of which were treated at 2 levels, and 4 at 3 levels. Patients wore a Lumboflex brace for 6 to 10 weeks afterwards. Good and excellent results were noted in 75%. There were no serious complications observed. Six cases had to be operated on later. In one third of the cases, pain yielded only after 3 to 4 months.

Three major disadvantages of chemonucleolysis are to be taken into account:

1. Hyperergic reactions against chymopapain.
2. The transient rise of pressure in the disc.
3. Sometimes the long time period before the method lends to a clinical success.

The positive effect depends on reduction of pressure in the nucleus pulposus and, subsequently, the adjacent protruded cartilage. Extraction of cartilage by instruments therefore should be superior.

In this respect, we began one year ago with percutaneous discectomy as published by Kambin [1–3], and 6 months ago with the nucleotome procedure according to Maroon [4] and Onik [5]. In the view of orthopedic surgeons, the following indications seem to be convincing for percutaneous discectomy:

1. Severe recurrent attacks of lumbalgia or lumboischialgia.
2. Resistance to conservative treatment over 4 to 6 weeks.
3. Minor neurologic symptoms such as Lasègue sign, reflex difference, sensible deficits.
4. Protrusion or prolapse on computer tomography, myelography or magnetic resonance imaging. The cartilage should not protrude more than one third into the spinal channel as a rule.
5. Correspondence of clinical symptoms and picture.

[1] Krankenhaus am Urban, Abteilung Orthopädie, Dieffenbachstr. 1, 1000 Berlin 61, FRG

Percutaneous Lumbar Discectomy
Ed. by H. M. Mayer and M. Brock

Relative contraindication can be seen in:

Severe spondylochondrosis, spinal stenosis, spondylolisthesis, and hypertrophic spondylarthrosis with narrowing of foramina.

Strict contraindications can be seen in:

1. Free fragments, massive prolapse.
2. Severe neurological deficit, motor paresis, bowel or bladder paresis.
3. Spondylitis or discitis.
4. Previous operation in the same level.
5. General contraindications.

We prefer the following procedure:

Using local anesthesia, the patient lies in a lateral scoliotic and kyphotic position. If the intervertebral space is wider than 3 mm, we introduce the tube of 4 to 5 mm over a trocar under control of an x-ray amplifier.

With special tongs, we are able to extract 2 to 3 g of cartilage. This usually takes 15 to 30 minutes. If the intervertebral space is smaller than 3 mm, we introduce the nucleotome of Maroon [4] and Onik [5] and extract automatically the same amount of tissue. In the lumbosacral level in most cases, we prefer the nucleotome of Maroon [4] and Onik [5] for anatomic reasons. Only in those cases in which the tubes of both methods cannot be introduced we perform chemonucleolysis.

Usually the patient leaves the hospital in the same evening or on the following day. A brace is given in cases of severe pain or instability.

The results in 18 cases of percutaneous discectomy and 14 cases of nucleotome treatment show that improvement has been seen in 70%. Three cases had to be operated on later because of a prolapse, one because of transient irritation of L 5.

Summary

In our hospital, chemonucleolysis has been widely replaced by percutaneous discectomy, but discectomy does not take the place of conventional operation. These new methods close the gap between cases which are conservatively no longer or operatively not yet to be treated. Further experience will show if this optimistic standpoint is justifiable.

References

1. Kambin P (1987) Mechanism of pain relief and research aspect of annular fenestration and percutaneous discectomy. International Symposium of Percutaneous Discectomy, Philadelphia, USA, March 1987
2. Kambin P, Gellman H (1983) Percutaneous lateral discectomy of the lumbar spine. Clin Orth Rel Res 174:127–132

3. Kambin P, Sampson S (1986) Posterolateral percutaneous suction-excision of herniated lumbar intervertebral disc. Clin Orth Rel Res 207: 27–43
4. Maroon JC, Onik G (1987) Percutaneous automated discectomy; a new method for lumbar disc removal. J Neurosurg 66: 143–146
5. Onik G et al. (1987) Automated percutaneous discectomy: Initial patient experience. Radiology 162/1: 129–132

Early Experience with Percutaneous Lateral Discectomy

M. B. STERN [1]

Abstract

Twenty-one patients are reported who underwent percutaneous lumbar discectomy for a herniated disc and sciatica. The criteria for inclusion in this series included: (1) a protruding disc in the lumbar area causing neural compression; (2) persistent sciatica; (3) failure of conservative treatment; (4) MRI, CT, or myelographic confirmation of the protrusion; (5) chronic low back pain with definite evidence of a protruding disc at the appropriate level. The only contraindication to the procedure is the presence of an extruded fragment. There were twelve males and nine females with an average age of 40. The operation is performed under local anesthesia and by the method of Kambin [3–6]. Twelve cases were at the L4–L5 level, eight were at the L5–S1 level, four were at the L3–L4 level, and one was at the L2–L3 level. Seventeen of 21 patients were relieved of their symptoms. One case was aborted due to inability to pass the cannula beneath arthritic facet joints. One complication occurred early while we were using general anesthetic. We injured an L5 nerve root causing a permanent foot drop. Major possible complications include: (1) infection; (2) nerve root injury: (3) vascular injury. A success rate of 85% is reported.

Percutaneous lateral discectomy is becoming an accepted alternative to lumbar laminectomy for protruding or herniated intervertebral discs in a select group of patients. The initial development of this procedure was by Dr. Sadhisa Hijikata [1] in Japan in 1975, and since that time Schreiber and Suzeawa [7], Hoppenfeld [2], and Kambin [3–6] have made the procedure more popular in the United States and elsewhere.

All authors stress in their papers that the most important point in the success of the procedure is the proper selection of patients. The criteria that must be met in order to consider a patient a candidate for this procedure are:

1. A protruding disc in the lumbar area causing neural compression.
2. Persistent sciatica.
3. Failure of conservative treatment consisting of bedrest, heat, analgesics, anti-inflammatorics, physical therapy, and epidural injections.
4. MRI, CT scan, or myelographic confirmation of the protrusion.

[1] Cedars-Sinai Medical Center, Department of Orthopedic Surgery, Los Angeles, CA 90048, USA

Percutaneous Lumbar Discectomy
Ed. by H. M. Mayer and M. Brock

5. Chronic low back pain with definite evidence of a protruding disc at the appropriate level.

The major contraindication to this procedure is evidence of an extruded disc fragment. A second contraindication in some centers has been an L 5–S 1 lesion, due to the difficulty of entering the disc space. In the general experience, however, this does not appear to be a problem in a majority of cases.

I present here a series of 21 patients who underwent percutaneous nucleotomy (Table 1). There were twelve males and nine females ranging in age from 23 years to 89 years, with an average age of 40 years. Follow-up was from one month to 20 months, with an average follow-up of 10.7 months. All of the patients fulfilled the above criteria, and four patients had the procedure performed at two levels simultaneously. All had clinical and radiological documentation of a significantly protruding disc with neural impingement (Figure 1). All had conservative treatment of at least two months duration consisting of bed rest, heat, anti-inflammatories, analgesics, and epidural injections without significant relief of their symptoms.

During this period of time 100 patients with low back pain and sciatica were seen and treated. On the regime described above, 70 patients improved, nine patients had a laminectomy (since they were not considered candidates for this procedure), and 21 did not improve and then were considered candidates for this procedure and form the basis of this paper.

There was failure of this procedure and subsequent laminectomy in three patients. One had the classical symptoms of low back pain and left sciatica, and a MRI showed marked protrusion at the L 4–L 5 and L 5–S 1 disc levels on the

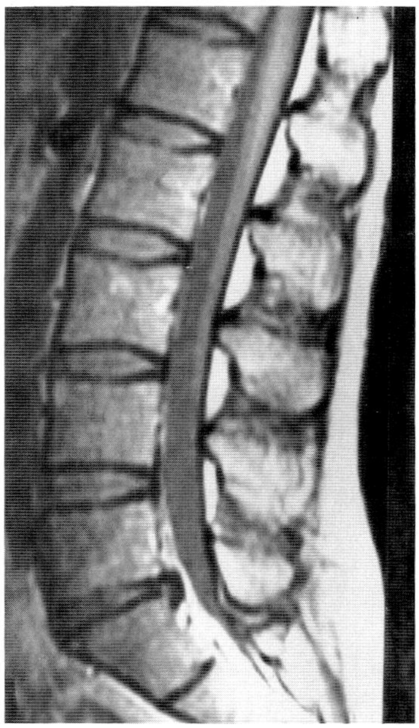

Fig. 1. MRI showing disc protrusion at L 5–S 1

Table 1. Patients' symptoms, findings and results

Name	Age	Sex	Symptoms	Myelogram, CT, MRI	Level	Follow-up	Results
S.R.	43	M	Low back pain, left sciatica, left ankle jerk, decreased sensation to left calf and foot.	MRI: Large disc protrusion on left	L5–S1	18 months (1/21/87)	E
J.R.	68	M	Severe spinal stenosis at L3–L4 and L4–L5 due to disc protrusion and arthritic changes. Left drop foot.	MRI: Severe spinal stenosis with significant disc protrusion	L3–L4 L4–L5	18 months (1/23/87)	E
M.D.	23	F	Low back pain and severe sciatica. Muscle power left foot, ankle jerk on left, and sensation left foot decreased.	MRI: Large protruding disc on left	L4–L5	9 months (10/12/87)	E
S.H.	25	M	Pain low back and right leg one year. Decreased range of motion of lumbosacral spine. Muscle strength of right foot and sensation of calf and foot decreased.	CT scan: Disc protrusion on right	L5–S1	13 months (6/29/87)	E
J.M.	36	M	Severe low back pain and left leg pain. Muscle power of left foot decreased. Sensation decreased on plantar left foot.	MRI: Large disc on left	L5–S1	8 months (12/3/87)	E
C.G.		F	Severe low back pain and left sciatica. Previous surgery at L4–L5. Post-op drop foot. No sciatica.	MRI: Disc protrusion	L4–L5	15 months	E
J.D.	66	F	Severe low back pain and right sciatica.	MRI: Severe disc protrusion	L3–L4	19 months (12/30/86)	E
H.T.	29	M	Low back pain and left sciatica. Sensation decreased in left calf and foot. Nucleotomy failed and 10 days later had laminectomy.	CT scan: Protrusions at MRI: Persistent protrusion at	L4–L5 L5–S1 L4–L5 L5–S1	14 months (5/16/87)	F
R.D.		M	Low back pain and left sciatica. Arthritic changes.	MRI: Disc protrusion on left	L5–S1	14 months	Aborted

T.K.	34	M	Severe low back pain and left sciatica. Normal neurological. 5 days post-nucleotomy severe pain in left leg.	CT scan and myelogram: Large disc on left. Repeat MRI: Extruded fragment	L4–L5 L4–L5	15 months (4/15/87)	F
A.P.	63	F	Severe low back pain radiating into both legs.	Myelogram and CT scan: Bulging discs	L3–L4 L4–L5	8 months (11/6/87)	E
S.P.	27	M	Severe low back pain and left leg pain.	MRI: Herniated disc with pressure on left L5 nerve root	L4–L5	9 months (11/10/87)	E
F.F.	45	M	Severe low back pain and right leg pain. Previous laminectomy at L4–L5 14 years ago.	MRI: Large disc protrusion on right	L4–L5	13 months (6/30/87)	E
E.C.	35	F	Severe low back pain and left leg pain.	Myelogram: Protrusion on left	L5–S1	17 months (3/3/87)	E
C.L.	67	F	Severe low back pain and right groin pain.	MRI: Large bulging disc on right	L2–L3	9 months (10/3/87)	E
W.G.	89	M	Severe low back pain and right sciatica.	MRI: Severe spinal stenosis with herniated disc	L3–L4	13 months (6/27/87)	E
D.S.	50	F	Severe low back pain and left sciatica.	Myelogram: Bulge	L4–L5	7 months (1/2/88)	E
M.L.	67	M	Severe low back pain and left sciatica. Initially successful but disc extruded following auto accident.	MRI: L5–S1 bulge	L5–S1	3 months (4/1/88)	E
S.C.	24	M	Industrial accident. Severe pain low back and left leg for 6 months.	MRI: L4–L5 bulge L5–S1 bulge	L4–L5 L5–S1	3 months (4/13/88)	F
D.S.	45	F	Severe low back pain and left sciatica.	MRI: Showing a large bulge	L4–L5	1 month (6/30/88)	E
K.R.	35	F	Severe low back pain and left leg pain.	MRI: Moderate protrusion	L4–L5	1 month (7/15/88)	E

left side with neural impingement. However, following a satisfactory two-level percutaneous discectomy, the patient improved for approximately one week and then began to have symptoms again of the same severity. He underwent lumbar laminectomy with disc removal at both these levels and was totally relieved of his symptoms by this operation.

One patient, following failure of the percutaneous discectomy to relieve his symptoms, had a second MRI which showed an extruded fragment at the same level. This was not present on his initial CT scan; it was confirmed at surgery. The patient underwent laminectomy and disc excision and is totally asymptomatic at this time.

A third patient had a successful percutaneous nucleotomy at L4–L5 and L5–S1 with relief of symptoms for one week, and then had a recurrence of left leg pain which was just as severe as before. He underwent a lumbar laminectomy at both levels with relief of symptoms.

A fourth patient had severe arthritic changes at the L5–S1 interspace, and the procedure was aborted following satisfactory placement of the spinal needle when the instrumentation would not pass severely arthritic facet joints at L5–S1. This patient subsequently underwent lumbar laminectomy and is asymptomatic at this time. He is not included in the follow-up studies.

Operative Procedure

I have performed percutaneous lumbar discectomy according to the description of Kambin. This is a procedure that was first described by Hijikada, later modified by Schreiber, and modified further by Kambin. I do not use a motorized nucleotome. No antibiotics were given in the first 17 cases.

The patient is in a prone position under Versed and fentanyl analgesia. We have simultaneous fluoroscopic capability in both the AP and lateral positions. Using one percent xylocaine in the skin, an 18-gauge spinal needle is started at a point 8 to 10 centimeters lateral to the midline in a position parallel to the abnormal disc space. The disc space is entered on the symptomatic side. Under fluoroscopic control, the needle is inserted into the appropriate disc space. Through this needle a 0.031 Kirschner wire is placed in the disc space and the needle removed. A one-inch incision is then made around the Kirschner wire and a dull pointed cannulated trochar is then inserted over the K-wire to the disc space.

A 6-millimeter cannula is then placed over the trocar again to the annulus and its position verified by fluoroscopy. Then the K-wire and dull trocar are removed. It is extremely important to state that pressure must be maintained against the 6-millimeter cannula to keep it abutting against the annulus fibrosus.

A 2-millimeter cutting instrument is then placed in the cannula and a hole is made in the annulus (Fig. 2). It is at this point that the patient may need a little more analgesia because this portion of the procedure is painful.

The 2-millimeter cutter is removed and a 4-millimeter cutter inserted and a 4-millimeter hole is made in the annulus. Under fluoroscopic control a pituitary

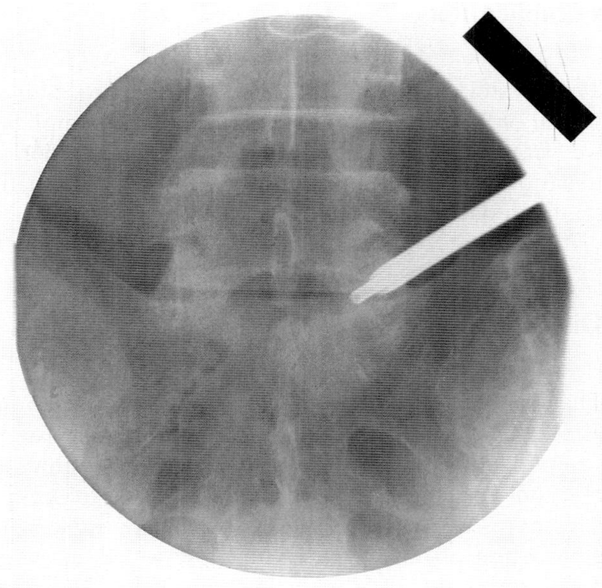

Fig. 2. X-ray showing cannula and cutter at L5–S1 interspace

rongeur is placed down the cannula, and 2 to 4 grams of disc removed. The 4-millimeter cutter is then placed down the cannula and a 50-cc syringe attached to it. Suction is applied until a loud pop is heard as the plunger is pulled up and out of the barrel. The pituitary rongeur is then replaced into the disc space and further disc is removed. Once sufficient disc has been removed, the cannula is removed and two sutures close the wound.

The patient is up that afternoon and discharged the following day.

Results

Twenty-one patients underwent percutaneous lumbar discectomy and 25 disc spaces were decompressed. Four patients had 2 levels done simultaneously. Twelve cases were at L4–L5, 8 cases at L5–S1, 4 at L3–L4, and one case was at L2–L3. From our 21 cases we excluded the one that we aborted at L5–S1 due to arthritic changes. Therefore, we had 17 of 20 patients who were relieved of their symptoms of sciatic pain and neurological findings of drop foot, weakness of toe extensors, and hypalgesia. All have returned to normal lives. This is a success rate of approximately 85% in a small series of cases.

Complications

The possible major complications of the procedure are disc space infection or neural or vascular injury. We have had one complication early in the series when we were using general anesthesia. We injured a nerve root causing a post-operative foot drop which 11 months later is still present. The patient, however, has no sciatica post-operatively.

Discussion

The idea of decompressing a lumbar disc space and relieving sciatica by an alternate route other than by lumbar laminectomy is not new. The possible complications that may ensue following traditional decompression via laminectomy and discectomy have caused surgeons to seek other less invasive ways of decompressing a pathological disc. There appears to be an ever-increasing accumulation of data from around the world, showing that percutaneous lateral discectomy being used in the appropriately selected cases and by surgeons trained in this technique, may help between 60–80% of these patients. If, however, the procedure does not succeed and the patient remains symptomatic, then the success of conventional lumbar laminectomy has not been jeopardized.

It is my impression that percutaneous lateral discectomy is an excellent procedure and should be considered as a form of conservative treatment for unremitting low back pain and sciatica caused by a protruding disc when all other forms of conservative treatment have failed and laminectomy is being considered.

References

1. Hijikata SA (1975) A method of percutaneous nuclear extraction. J Toden Hospital 5:39
2. Hoppenfeld S (1983) Percutaneous removal of herniated lumbar disc through the tube technique. Presented at the Association of Bone and Joint Surgeons, Sea Island, Georgia, May 1983
3. Kambin P, Breger MD (1987) Percutaneous lateral discectomy: Anatomy and mechanism. Clin Orthop 223:145
4. Kambin P, Gellman H (1983) Percutaneous lateral discectomy of the lumbar spine: A preliminary report. Clin Orthop 174:127
5. Kambin P, Sampson S (1984) Laminectomy vs. percutaneous lateral discectomy: A comparative study. Orthop Trans 8:408
6. Kambin P, Sampson S (1986) Posterior lateral percutaneous suction excision of herniated intervertebral discs: Report of interim results. Clin Orthop 207:37
7. Schreiber A, Suezawa Y (1986) Transdiscoscopic percutaneous nucleotomy in disc herniation. Orthop Rev 15:75

Automated Percutaneous Lumbar Discectomy (APLD)

Early Results of Automated Percutaneous Lumbar Discectomy

H.-P. KAPS and H. COTTA [1]

Introduction

Percutaneous discectomy for noninvasive treatment of the herniated lumbar disc is of growing interest. The new technique avoids several risks of traditional therapy, i.e. surgical disc removal by laminectomy. Percutaneous discectomy was first performed by Hijikata [1] and in Switzerland by Suezawa and Rüttimann [3], removing disc material with a long pituitary forceps through a posterolateral approach.

Methods

Since January 1988, physicians in the Orthopedic Clinic of the University of Heidelberg have used the technique described by Onik [2]; the so-called automated percutaneous lumbar discectomy (APLD). The nucleus pulposus is aspirated by a dorsolateral approach to the disc space with a 2-mm aspiration probe under local anesthesia. The probe is positioned under C-arm fluoroscopic control in two planes.

The criteria for patient selection are disc protrusion and herniated nucleus pulposus in an area consistent with the specific clinical findings. There should be a major complaint of sciatica American authors report in first publications about success rates of 70–90%, removing 2 g of disc material on average.

Results

We report about our own results of 67 patients treated by the APLD from January to June 1988.

In two patients, APLD was not possible because of permanent radicular pain while trying to puncture the disc (disc level L4–L5 and L5–S1). In two other cases, the disc level was reached by the probe, but no material could be aspirated (Sicca aspiration).

[1] Orthopädische Universitätsklinik, Schlierbacher Landstr. 200a, 6900 Heidelberg, FRG

Percutaneous Lumbar Discectomy
Ed. by H. M. Mayer and M. Brock

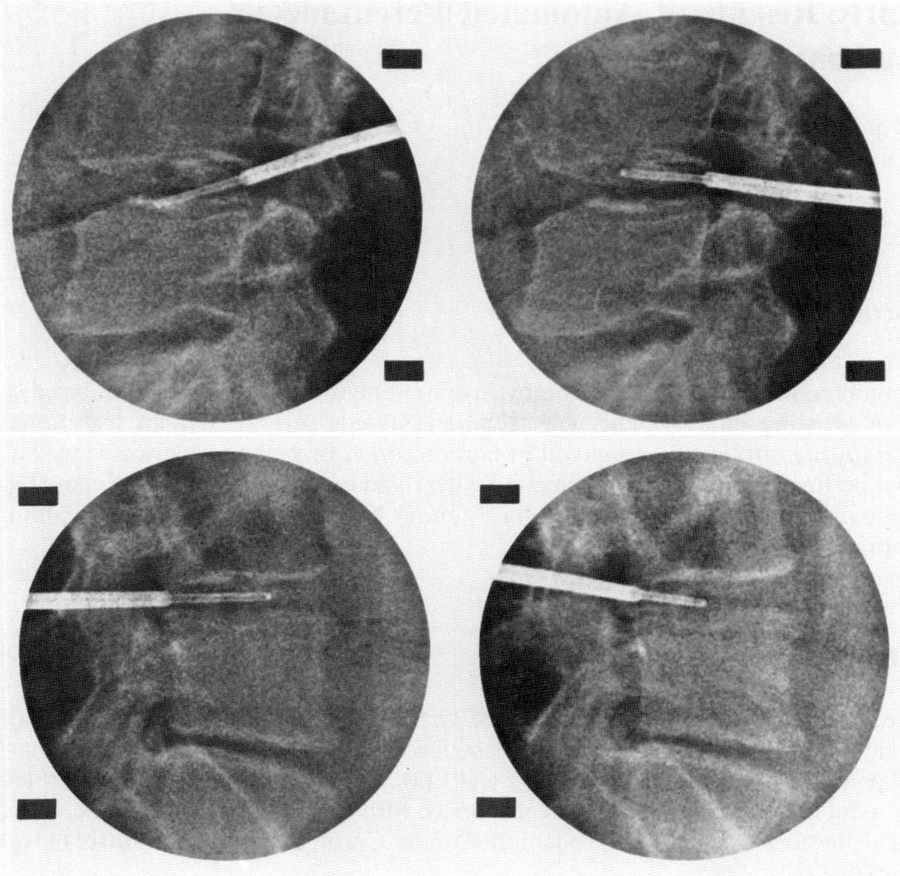

Fig. 1. Tip of the probe reaches a large proportion of the disc space by being moved in different planes

We routinely use the straight and flexed trocar in all disc levels. Figure 1 demonstrates that by moving the nucleotome up and down or parallel to the disc space, nearly the whole disc space can be reached by the probe.

Patient demographics are shown in Table 1. Forty-four of the nucleotome procedures were performed at the level L 4–L 5, 22 at the level L 5–S 1, one at the level L 5–L 6, and two combined on level L 3–L 4 and L 4–L 5. We have been successful in 82% of all cases (55 of 67), with 22 patients (33%) completely recovered. Forty-nine patient showed a partial recovery and 18 patients failed. Seventy-three percent had been satisfied after the procedure.

Table 2 demonstrates that the best results are found in mere sciatica (leg pain greater than back pain).

The average postoperative hospital stay was 4 days, the average working time of the probe 20 min, and 3 g of disc material were removed on average.

Table 1. Patient demographics

67 patients	69 disc levels
average age	41 years (17–68)
males 50	females 17
postoperative days	4 days (1–28)
operation time	20 min (10–30)
removed disc material	3 grs. (0,5–5)

Table 2. Results in APLD of 50 cases with leg pain and 17 cases with back pain

	Complete	Partial	None
leg pain (n=50)	18 (36%)	24 (48%)	8 (16%)
back pain (n=17)	4 (24%)	9 (52%)	4 (24%)
total (n=67)	22 (33%)	33 (49%)	12 (18%)

Recovery from paresis was recorded in 14 of 28 cases and from sensation loss in 20 of 27 cases.

In combination with relative spinal stenosis, 5 patients recovered completely, 6 partially, and only one did not recover. In contrast, only 3 of 17 patients with severe degenerative changes improved completely, 13 partially, and one did not recover. Most of the patients of the last group had more back pain than leg pain.

Subsequent open surgery followed in 9 patients with previous APLD. All cases showed a little free fragment that had not been recognized in the CT scan. In conclusion, from our short experience of APLD we postulate the following:

Indications

Good indications
Leg pain

- neurologic findings in a specific dermatomal distribution
- positive straight leg raising test
- positive CT scan consistent with clinical findings

Relative contraindications
Leg pain

- degenerative facet disease
- relative stenosis of recessus lateralis or spinal canal
- previous surgery of the same segment

Absolute contraindications
Leg pain

- free fragment
- absolute spinal stenosis

Mechanical low back pain (pseudoradicular pain)
Lumbar pain only.

References

1. Hijikata SA, Yamagishi M, Nakayama T, Oomori K (1975) Percutaneous discectomy – a new treatment method for lumbar disc herniation. J Toden Hosp 5:39
2. Onik G, Helms CA, Ginsburg L, Hoaglund FT, Morris J (1985) Percutaneous lumbar discectomy using a new aspiration probe. AJNR 6:290–293
3. Suezawa Y, Rüttimann B (1983) Indikation, Methodik und Ergebnisse der perkutanen Nukleotomie bei lumbaler Diskushernie. Z Orthop 121:25

Automated Percutaneous Lumbar Discectomy (APLD)

R. CARTOLARI, P. DAVIDOVITS, and M. GAGLIARDELLI [1]

Introduction

The Onik Nucleotome System achieves less traumatic surgery in patients with lumbar disc protrusion [3, 4].

Indications

The main indications are subannular disc herniations. The most important parameters for patient selection are:

1. monolateral or bilateral lumbar and/or sciatic pain with precise dermatomal distribution
2. paresthesia with precise dermatomal distribution
3. positive Lasègue test
4. CT confirmation of disc protrusion at the level corresponding to the peripheral symptomatology
5. symptoms persisting after at least six weeks of conservative therapy.

Contraindications

1. Degenerative facet disease
2. Spinal stenosis
3. CT findings of free fragments into the spinal canal.

Materials and Methods

From July 1987 to March 1988, we performed in our center 27 automated percutaneous lumbar discectomies (APLD) in 24 patients (19 at L 4/L 5, 8 at L 5/S 1).

[1] Centro Medico Italiano, Gruppo Hesperia Sanita, Viale Filopanti 12, 40126 Bologna, Italy

Percutaneous Lumbar Discectomy
Ed. by H. M. Mayer and M. Brock

One patient underwent APLD twice at the same level because of recurrent symptoms. Two patients underwent APLD at both levels in the same session. 23 patients had a central or posterolateral disc protrusion, one of them had undergone conventional spinal surgery three times before. One patient had intra-foraminal disc herniation.

Before APLD, X-rays of the lumbar spine had been taken in all patients. CT examination from L3 to S1 and some CT scans in a prone position at the level of herniation were performed to localize the position of the intestinal tract.

Some authors suggest the necessity of a preoperative discography to verify the continuity of the annulus fibers. We believe that the introduction of any substance inside the disc space increases the risk of infection. Thus, in our opinion, discography should be limited only to those cases in which, at CT, disc protrusion is so great that a high probability of a real expulsion of the hernia exists. Similarly, preoperative myelography should be performed only in particular and selected patients.

Technique

With the patient in a prone position, the disc space is identified by intermittent biplanar fluoroscopic control. In local anesthesia, we reach the disc with the trocar from a posterolateral approach (about 10 cm from the midline) [1, 2]. General anesthesia is contraindicated. When the disc surface is reached (a typical "elastic" resistance is felt), the tip of the trocar should be on lateral view at the level of the posterior vertebral body line and on AP view at the level of the lateral vertebral body line. If the patient experiences any sign of radicular irritation, the trocar must be retracted and re-directed.

1 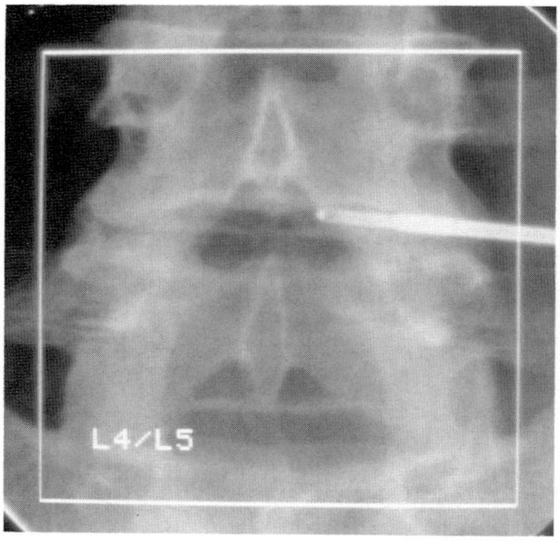

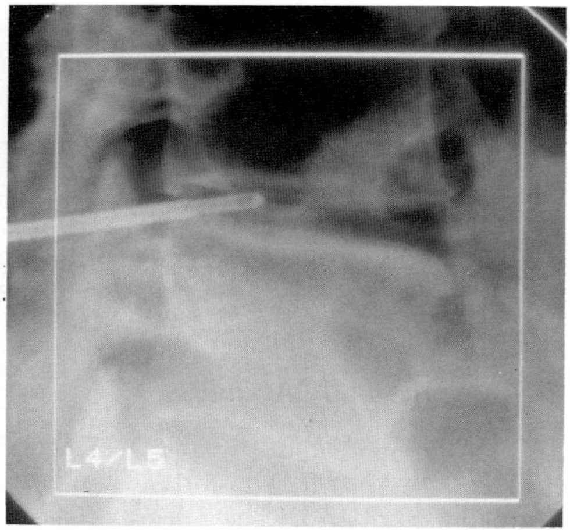 2

Fig. 1. AP view of nucleotome probe positioned in L4/L5 discal space

Fig. 2. Lateral view of probe in same patient

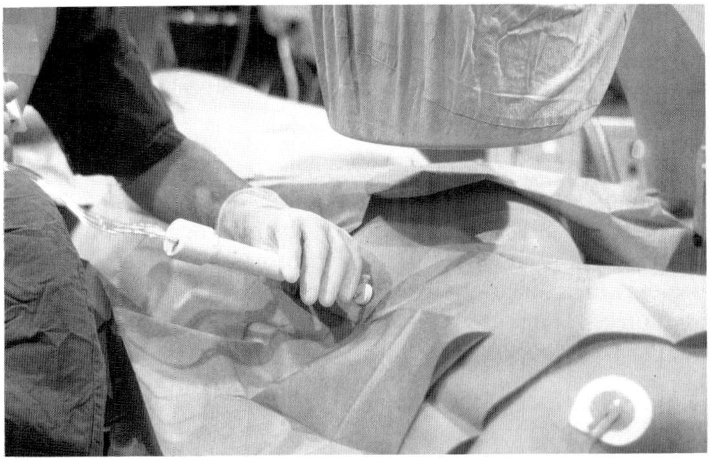

Fig. 3. General view of patient in prone position on operating table

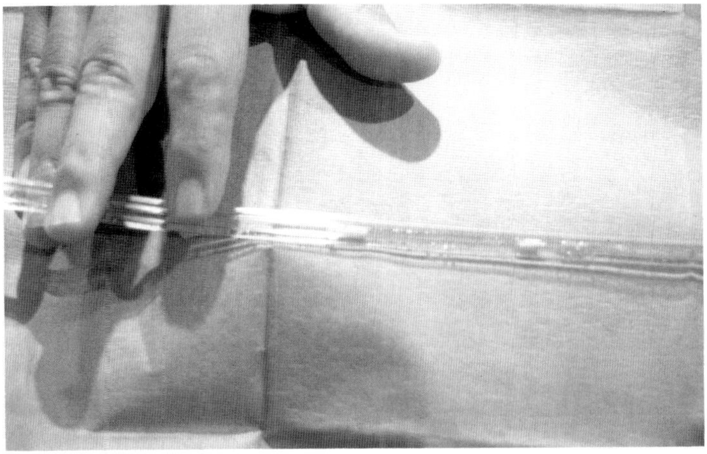

Fig. 4. Disc fragments during aspiration

When the trocar is introduced into the disc, in the lateral view its tip should be localized in the center; in AP view the tip should project between the pedicles. Using the trocar as a guide, the cannula and the dilatator are inserted. Incision of annulus is made by a trephine placed over the trocar and through the cannula. When annulus is incised, trocar and trephine are removed, leaving the cannula in place. On this guide, the nucleotome probe is inserted inside the disc (Figs. 1–3). At this time, the cutting-aspiration procedure begins (Fig. 4); time needed usually varies from 35 to 50 minutes. APLD ends when at least 2.5–4 grams of material have been aspirated; probe and cannula are extracted simultaneously. All patients were released on the second or third postoperative day. They should keep bed-rest for 7 days and receive an antibiotic prophylaxis for a period of 5 days. We recommend an orthopedic cast for one month and, for the same period, the patient should refrain from any heavy physical exercise.

Results

20 patients fully recovered, 19 of them returned to a normal social life within 40 days and are free from any symptoms. Two patients had no variation in the pre-existing clinical picture. One of them underwent conventional laminectomy, and a free fragment was then found. The previously operated patient had partial recovery (Table 1).

Table 1. Results

Patient	Level		Follow-up (months)	Compli-cations	Results	
	L4/L5	L5/S1			Good	Poor
1. G.S.″	×		12		×	
2. M.N.′		×	1			× (f.f.)
3. P.M.		×	12		×	
4. R.G.	×		11		×	
5. M.G.		×	2			×
M.G.		×	10	NRI	×	
6. T.G.	×		11		×	
7. P.L.″	×		10		×	
8. N.M.	×		10		×	
9. F.G.′	×		10			×
10. S.M.″	×		10	LBP	×	
11. F.F.	×		10		×	
12. P.R.	×		9		×	
13. D.G.		×	9		×	
14. S.F.	×		9		×	
15. T.M.″	×		9		×	
16. P.F.		×	9		×	
17. R.C.	×		9		×	
18. T.P.	×		8		×	
19. M.D.	×		8		×	
20. S.B.″	×	×	7		×	
21. M.F.‴	×		6			
22. T.L.″	×		6		×	
23. A.F.	×	×	4	D		
24. F.F.		×	4		×	

Key to symbols: ′ = no variation in symptoms; ″ = transitory low back pain; ‴ = previously operated patient; NRI = nerve root irritation; LBP = severe low back pain; D = discitis; f.f. = free fragment into spinal canal.

Complications

The major complication was discitis. One of the patients who underwent APLD at two levels (L 4/5 and L 5/S 1) developed L 5/S 1 discitis. The patient who underwent APLD twice at the same level developed a temporary radicular irritation of the L 5 root after the second APLD, probably caused by the approach maneuvers. This disappeared after 40 days with complete restitutio ad integrum. Six patients hads light to severe postoperative low back pain at the site of APLD: In five of them, this pain disappeared within 15 to 30 days. In the sixth, severe pain continued for over 90 days and less intensely for a further period of 60 days.

In most of these patients [5], we positioned the trocar and the cannula twice in order to obtain a sufficient quantity of disc material. We believe that the consequent "discal stress" was the temporary cause of this pain.

Follow-Up

In all patients, clinical and CT controls were performed. CT controls were made about two months after APLD. In patients with full recovery, CT showed pictures varying from complete absence to complete persistence of disc protrusion.

As a general rule, CT "improvement" was in inverse ratio with the "age" of symptoms: the shorter the time of sciatic pain before APLD, the better the CT improvement. We believe this could be in relation with reduced Sharpey fiber elasticity. A confirmation of this hypothesis came from the multi-surgery patient. When this patient came to us for observation, his lumbar spine had been stabilized with Harrington's rods. From a clinical point of view, he had sciatic pain corresponding to a nerve root. Pre-APLD CT and myelography showed disc protrusion at the L 4/L 5 level. After APLD the patient had partial recovery with resolution of L 4 root irritation.

Control CT showed a reduced L 4/L 5 protrusion. Persisting irritation of the L 5 root and, above all, intolerance to Harrington's rods led the patient to conventional surgery. On this occasion, scar tissue was found around the L 5 root. An exploration of the L 4/L 5 discal space showed a small soft disc protrusion without any sign of compression of dural sac and nerve roots. The disc was completely empty inside.

Conclusions

Even though our experience is still limited, we believe that APLD must be considered the first choice of surgical approach in any disc protrusion and a real alternative to conventional laminectomy in some selected, previously operated patients.

The follow-up is, above all, clinical. CT can, in fact, only show the protrusion of non-elastic, but not compressive, annulus fibers.

In cases of recurrent symptoms, there are no contraindications for a second APLD or conventional laminectomy.

Major complications such as discitis or permanent nerve root lesions can be avoided by complete asepsis and caution during disc approach maneuvers. Transitory lower back pain could be experienced by patients after APLD and should be referred to as "discal stress".

References

1. Hijikata S, Yamagishi M, Nakayama T, Ohmori K (1975) Percutaneous diskectomy. J Toden Hospital, 5:5–13
2. Hijikata S, Nakayama T, Ichihama M (1978) Percutaneous nucleotomy for low back pain. Rel. SICOT XIV World Congress, Kyoto, October 1978
3. Onik G, Helms CA, Ginsberg L, Hoaglund FT, Morris J (1985) Percutaneous lumbar diskectomy using a new aspiration probe: porcine and cadaver model. Radiology 155:251–252
4. Onik G, Maroon JC, Helms C, Schweigel J, Mooney V, Kahanovitz N, Day A, Morris J, McCulloch JA, Reicher M (1987) Automated percutaneous diskectomy: Initial patient experience. Radiology 162:129–132
5. Schreiber A, Suezawa Y (1986) Transdiscoscopic percutaneous nucleotomy in disk herniation. Orthop Rev XV, 1:75–78

Comparison of Chemonucleolysis with Chymopapain to Percutaneous Automated Discectomy: A Surgeon's First 50 Cases of Each

F. D. Cooney [1]

Abstract

The results of one surgeon's first 50 patients treated with chemonucleolysis with chymopapain are compared to the first 50 patients treated with percutaneous automated discectomy.

The use of chymopapain in nucleolysis of a herniated lumbar disc has been involved in controversy since its beginning, 24 years ago. Its utilization increased significantly and then stopped abruptly because of the realization of its complications. Ninety percent of all complications associated with the use of chymopapain in chemonucleolysis were associated with surgeons who had done ten or less procedures [3]. For this obvious reason, the complications of this drug are less when utilized in medical centers where considerably higher number of these procedures are performed. It is appropriate, therefore, to analyze one's first experience with any new surgical procedure. I will compare the efficacy and complications of my first 50 chemonucleolysis with chymopapain performed in 1983 to the first 50 cases of percutaneous automated discectomy performed since 1987. The recommended protocols for both of these different surgical procedures were followed in detail [1, 2].

Materials and Methods

The group treated with chymopapain were those patients who failed conservative measures consisting of at least 6 weeks of bed rest and medications, and who had sciatic pain due to a herniated disc demonstrated by myelography and CT scanning. Patients who were excluded were those who had a known sensitivity to papaya, those demonstrating spinal stenosis or spondylolisthesis, or those who had previous surgery at the proposed site of injection. Patients who demonstrated a positive Chymofast test, elevated sed. rate, or significant allergy history were excluded. Histamine receptor antagonists were prescribed preoperatively. The procedure was performed in the operating room with excellent fluoroscopy with an image intensifier under general anesthesia which was recommended at that time. Discograms were performed at that time and were all abnormal in the discs

[1] George Washington University School of Medicine, Washington Hospital Center, Washington, DC 20037, USA

Percutaneous Lumbar Discectomy
Ed. by H. M. Mayer and M. Brock

injected. During the procedure, the patient received a test dose of 0.3 ml of chymopapain. They were observed for 15 minutes; the injection of between 1.5 and 2 cc of chymopapain was administered by an 18 gauge, 6 in needle with the patient in the lateral position. Post-injection the patients received pain medications as needed. They remained hospitalized overnight and increased activity as their residual discomfort would allow.

All of our 50 percutaneous discectomies were performed with a 2 mm blunt-tipped suction/cutting probe (Nucleotome). These patients were treated under local anesthesia with the patient in the lateral position with fluoroscopic guidance. All had one-level surgery. There were 31 males and 19 females. Eight patients were done at L3–4, 35 patients were done at L4–5 and 7 patients were done at L5–S1. It is important to note that instrumentation to reach the L5–S1 disc space did not become available until early 1988.

Indications for surgery included those who failed to improve with the standard bed rest and medications for at least 6 weeks' duration and had radicular pain associated with a positive straight leg raising test. The pretreatment radiological workup included primarily plain films and MRI scans. In our practice, MRI scans have become the standard diagnostic test for herniated discs. Contraindications to the percutaneous procedure included insufficient nonoperative treatment; evidence of a sequestered and/or free fragment of disc and lumbar stenosis. Other contraindications are infection or other conditions which place the patient at risk, including poor fluoroscopic equipment. Previous surgery was not considered a contraindication.

Preoperative planning must rule out retroperitoneal structures that may be in the path of the trocar. Recent literature indicates that the colon may be displaced posteriorly in up to 4% of the patients and could be in the path of the trocar. A single non-magnified CT scan slice should be taken through the involved disc space to include the abdomen. This should be done with the patient in the prone position.

The discectomies were performed with the patient in the lateral position with the ipsilateral pain side superior. The entry point was usually 10–12 cm from the midline. The posterolateral approach is used to avoid the spinal canal and since he is awake, he can be monitored to avoid injuring the nerve root.

A series of larger instrumentation is introduced into the disc space. The aspiration probe or the Nucleotome is placed into the disc space through a 2.8 mm cannula. This probe is 8 inches long with a blunt tip and a single side port utilizing a guillotine suction-aspiration and cutting action. The disc material which is suspended in saline is aspirated through the inner cannula to a collection bottle. The usual aspirating cutting period would last approximately 30–45 minutes. More recently, we have been using shorter periods of aspiration because we have been utilizing the curved cannula, regardless of the level of disc.

All 50 of our patients were done on an outpatient basis. The procedure was performed in the Operating Room under local anesthesia. General anesthesia being contraindicated. There was no problem with bleeding in any of the cases. The patients went to the post-anesthesia recovery room and then were discharged home. They were allowed to return to work or school usually within the next few days.

Results (Figs. 1–5)

One must realize that in comparing these two procedures that more time has elapsed since the enzyme injections than our more recent percutaneous discectomies. The number of patients is small and the time elapsed is not long enough to judge absolute success or recurrences in the latter group. It is appropriate, however, to evaluate a surgeon's early experience with regard to complications, apparent successes and failures.

The results were classified as excellent in those patients who are pain free, back to work or school, and are on no medication. Good results are those patients that are having some pain, but are back to work or school and are taking no medication. Patients classified as fair are those who had some improvement and returned to work but felt the procedure was not of great benefit. Failures were those with no benefit.

As one sees in the comparison chart, both procedures successfully treated herniated lumbar discs with a 72% success rate with chymopapain and an 82% success rate with percutaneous discectomy. Patients with anaphylaxis were treated without any problem. There were no incidents of transverse myelitis. One patient had an L 5 nerve root injury second to needle insertion. This gradually improved over one year. There was one complete disc space destruction which was treated with steroids, but not antibiotics and classified as a chemical discitis. I have included as complications, significant back spasms lasting over 3 months which occurred in 46% of our chemonucleolysis patients. The percutaneous discectomy group was free of this episodes of spasms even one year post-injection. This side effect has never been registered as a complication of the procedure, but more or less has been listed as an expected result. Although it was the complica-

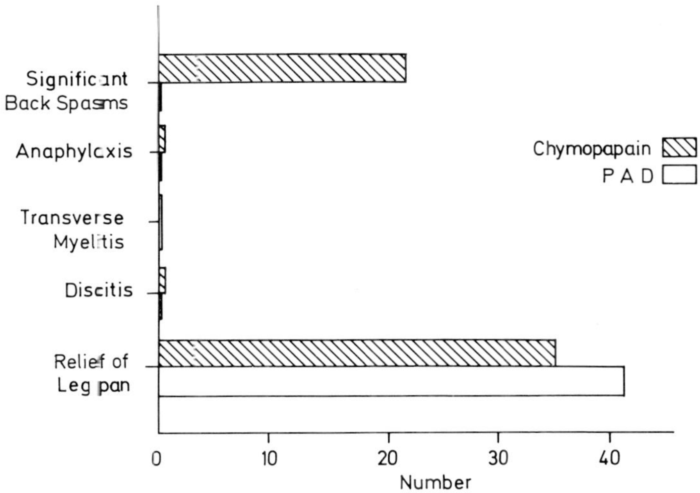

Fig. 1. The complications and success rate of chemonucleolysis with chymopapain compared to percutaneous automated discectomy

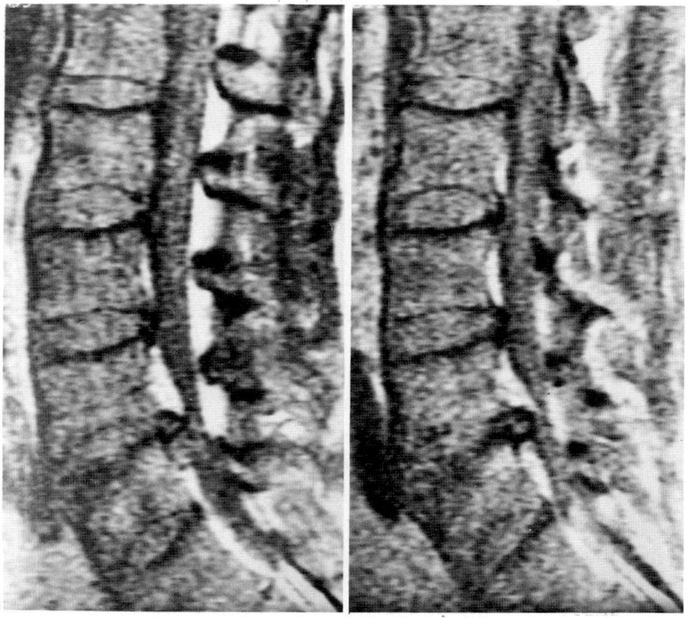

Fig. 2. 39-year-old male with back and left leg pain, sagittal MRI

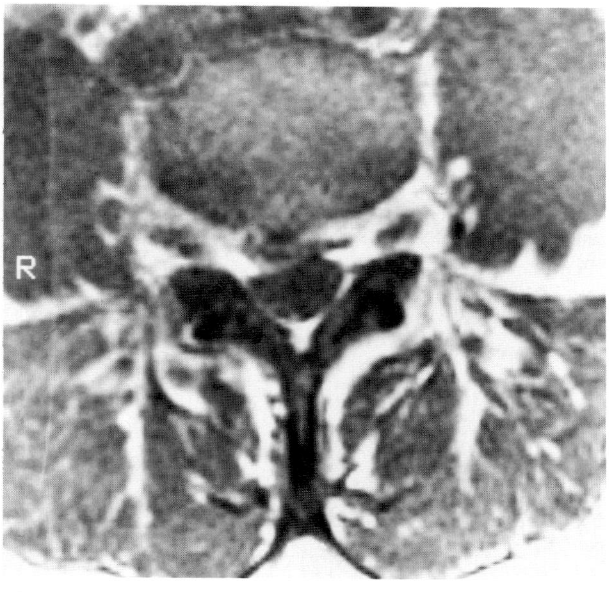

Fig. 3. 39-year-old male with back and left leg pain, axial MRI

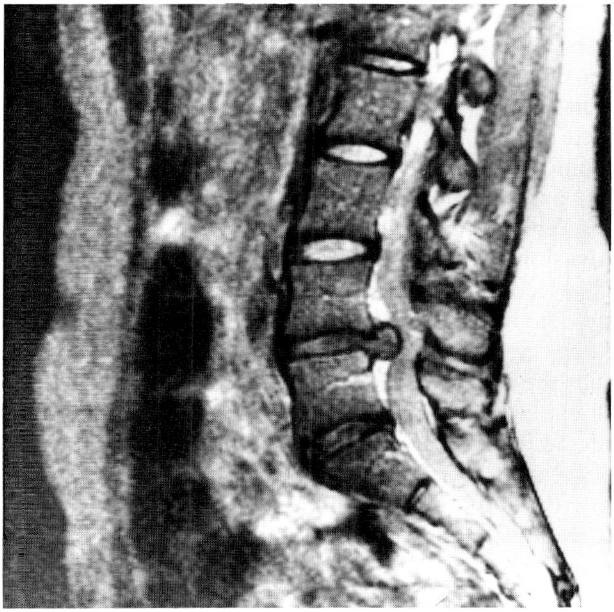

Fig. 4. 21-year-old female with back and bilateral leg pain, sagittal MRI

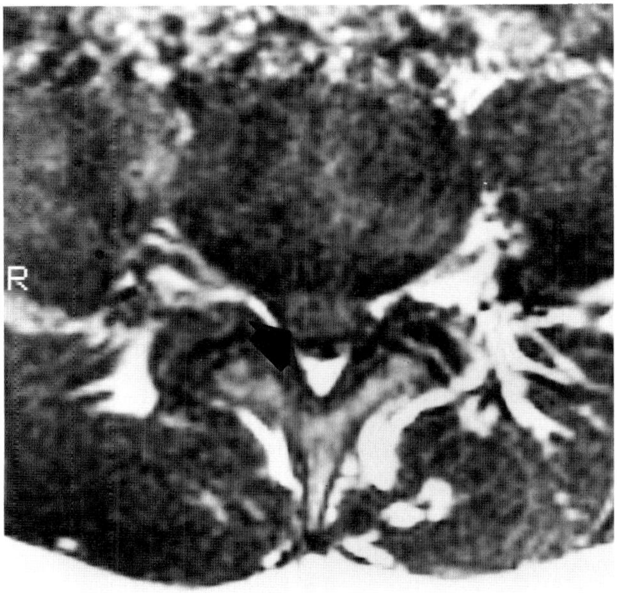

Fig. 5. 21-year-old female with back and bilateral leg pain, axial view

tion of transverse myelitis and the uproar in the press that practically ended this procedure in the United States, it was the persistent back spasms which was the most common source of dissatisfaction to the patients. Although it is my belief that chemonucleolysis with chymopapain certainly can be performed in specialized centers and the terrible complications of myelitis, hemorrhage and death would be significantly reduced and possibly completely avoided, the complication of back spasms will still significantly persist.

With percutaneous discectomy the primary advantage is that there is no invasion of the spinal canal and no postoperative intraspinal perineural scarring. The secondary advantage is the early return to full activity.

The amount of disc material removed from each patient was not compared; however, this data is still available to us. It is the author's personal impression that the result in percutaneous discectomy is not in proportion to the amount of disc material removed. Indeed, the procedure's primary relief may be in lowering of the intradiscal pressure and therefore subsequent decreased irritation of the nerve root. With this in mind, I have tried to enlarge the actual fenestration made into the annulus at the end of the procedure by moving the Nucleotome in various directions to cause the opening to increase in size. Also, a larger opening permits residual disc material to exit through the fenestration into the lateral paraspinal muscles, causing no clinical symptoms.

In conclusion, it has been my experience that both procedures effectively can relieve a patient of his radicular pain, and if chemonucleolysis with chymopapain is performed in specialized centers with greater experienced personnel, the serious side effects will be greatly diminished, but the back spasms, the most common undesirable effect, will persist. With automated percutaneous discectomy, the success rates seem to be equally good or better without any of the complications of the enzyme. In our practice, automated percutaneous discectomy is an appropriate adjunct and has replaced the use of chymopapain.

References

1. Javid MJ, Nordby EJ, Ford LT, Hejna WJ, Whisler WW, Burton C, Millett K et al. (1983) Safety and efficacy of chymopapain (Chymodiactin) in herniated nucleus pulposus with sciatica. JAMA 249: 2489–2494
2. Maroon JC, Onik G (1987) Percutaneous automated discectomy: a new method for lumbar disc removal. J Neurosurg 66: 143–146
3. Smith L (1988) First International Intradiscal Society Meeting, Fort Lauderdale/FL 1988 (Unpublished data)

Automated Percutaneous Nucleotomy by Pain Scale

G. Corkill, J. Kimple, and R. Corkill [1]

Introduction

Percutaneous automated nucleotomy promises to provide a valuable alternative to the patients with lumbar disc lesions in many, but not all, instances [1, 4, 5]. Since the initiation of this procedure by Onik and Maroon [3], this procedure has gained rapid acceptance, some 12000 procedures being carried out by April 1988. To evaluate the procedure's efficacy and the time course of pain relief following the procedure as the purpose of the present study, with special objective advising preoperative/postoperative patients.

Materials and Methods

21 patients consecutively seen for lower lumbar disc related radiculopathy underwent nucleotomy for low back pain and radiculopathy.

Postoperative management was by the regime described by Morris [2] involving mild analgesics for two weeks and progressive exercises for twelve weeks with a varying time of return to work depending on the back-stressing nature of the individual patient's employment.

Follow up was up to 134 days (range = 2–134)
(mean = 37.79)

Patients were asked to rate their leg and back pain on four occasions, preoperatively, in the immediate postoperative phase, in an intermediate postoperative time and on a final occasion. These postoperative scores were then converted to percent residual scores by comparison with the preoperative scores and treated statistically by T-test and R-test for improvement and correlation with the passage of time.

[1] North State Neurosurgery, 2252 Court Street, Redding, CA 96001, USA

Percutaneous Lumbar Discectomy
Ed. by H.M. Mayer and M. Brock

Table 1. Leg pain raw scores

Patient	Preoperative score	Immediate postoperative score	Intermediate postoperative score	Final postoperative score
1	7	0	0	0
2	6	0	0	0
3	8	4	3	0
4	10	0	0	0
5	5	1	1	1
6	7	6	1	0
7	8	0	6	3
8	7	1	2	2
9	3	1	1.5	3
10	9	0	0	0
11	8	7	7	6
12	8	6	6	4
13	7	8	6	6
14	4	0.5	0	0
15	8	3.5	5.5	4
16	7.5	4	3	1.5
17	5	1	5	0.5
18	7	2.5	4.4	3
19	8	–	1	0
20	8	–	2	3
21	6	–	3	–
Mean	6.976	2.527	2.733	1.85
T-test value	–	6.4521	6.829	9.066
P-value	–	<0.001	<0.001	<0.001

Table 2. Back pain raw scores

Patient	Preoperative score	Immediate postoperative score	Intermediate postoperative score	Final postoperative score
1	10	0	5	5
2	5	3	3.5	3
3	8	3	7.5	1
4	9	1	1.5	1.5
5	5	6	1	1
6	5	4	0	3
7	8	1	6	3
8	6	0	1	1
9	9	6	2	0
10	9	3	2.5	0
11	2	1	2	2
12	0	8	1	4
13	8	0.5	6	6
14	4	1	0.5	0.5
15	3	1	4	4
16	2	2	0	0

Table 2. (continued)

Patient	Preoperative score	Immediate postoperative score	Intermediate postoperative score	Final postoperative score
17	5	4	3	2
18	8.5	2.4	0	7.5
19	8	–	1.5	5
20	8	–	3.5	0
21	8	–	–	–
Mean	6.2142	2.6055	2.575	2.47
T-test value	–	4.479	4.721	4.9
P-value	–	<0.001	<0.001	<0.001

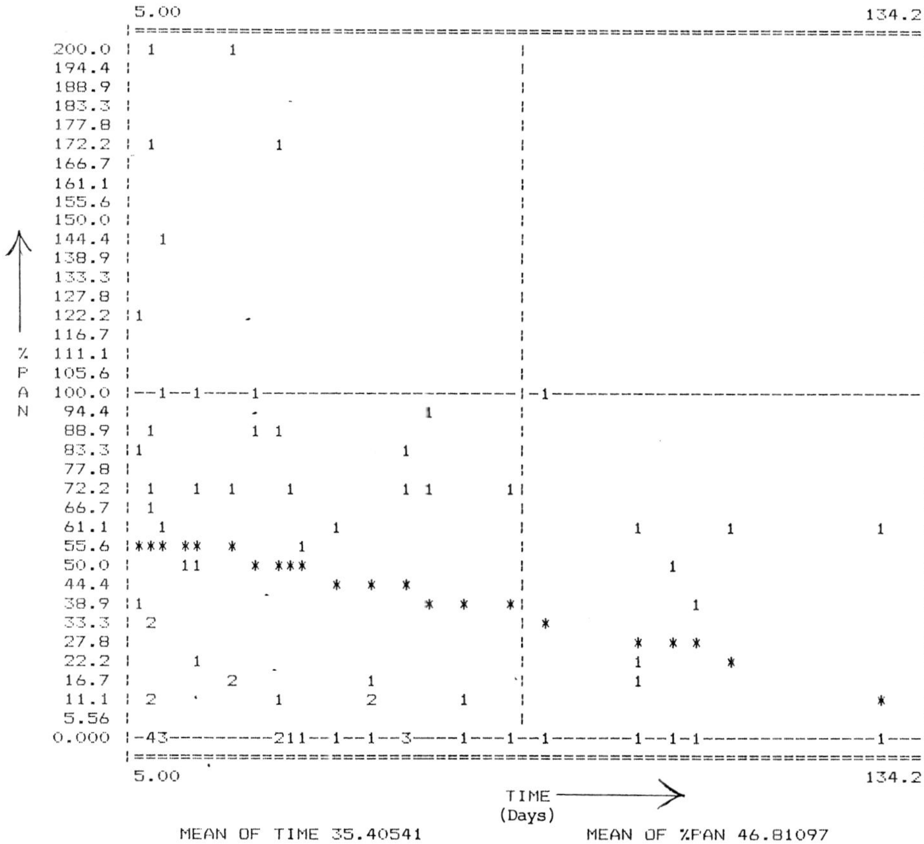


```
CORRELATION COEFFICIENT -     -0.2237005
T VALUE                 -     -2.0399
PROBABILITY             -     <0.05
```

Fig. 1. Postoperative interval residual percentage pain correlation (leg and back combined)

Results (Fig. 1, Tables 1, 2)

It was found that for both leg and back, there was marked improvement immediately which lessened to some extent in the intermediate postoperative phase and finally became even greater in terms of improvement in the final phase.

There was no morbidity or mortality. Two patients whose details are not shown are describable as surgical failures, their lumbosacral disc spaces having proved inaccessible to the nucleotome.

Discussion

The anatomy of disc prolapse implies that the posterior longitudinal ligament is initially distorted, following which the root contributing to the sciatic nerve is subsequently compressed and distorted. Reduction in the bulk of the disc would lead to improvement of leg pain before that of the back pain, as the sequence of compression is reversed. The results show greatest improvement values for the legs. Improvement with time, is of course, a feature of disc syndromes of many sorts, but in this study it appears to date from the nucleotomy, and to be maintained and relatively statistically significant in this group of postoperative patients. The increase in pain in the intermediate postoperative phase, may relate to cessation of pain medication as is called for in the postoperative regime.

Overall, this procedure appears effective when done for appropriate indications.

Acknowledgement. My sincere thanks to Wanda Attebery for preparation of this manuscript.

References

1. Friedman WA (1983) Percutaneous diskectomy: an alternative to chemonucleolysis. Neurosurgery 13: 542–547
2. Morris J (in press) Personal communication
3. Onik G, Maroon J (1987) Percutaneous automated diskectomy: a new method for lumbar disk removal. J Neurosurg 66: 143–146
4. Onik G, Helms C, Ginsburg L et al. (1985) Percutaneous lumbar diskectomy using a new aspiration probe: porcine and cadaver model. Radiology 155: 251–252
5. Onik G, Helms C, Ginsburg L et al. (1985) Percutaneous lumbar diskectomy using a new aspiration probe. AJNR 6: 290–293

Percutaneous Discectomy – Personal Observations of 27 Cases

S. M. REZAIAN and M. L. SILVER [1]

Introduction

It is now 60 years since the late Dr. Walter E. Dandy wrote the paper that called the attention of the medical world to the entity of herniation of the lumbar intervertebral disc [1]. From that time until the present, there has been a never-ending outpouring of papers giving details of surgical techniques used in the effort to correct the back and sciatic pain, associated with neurological involvement including motor weakness, sensory impairment, and reflex changes in the lower extremities, together with the varying responses of the patient to the modalities of treatment employed. Even so, few basic changes have emerged from all the papers on the surgical treatment of protruded lumbar discs.

However, the introduction of the present technique of percutaneous discectomy appears to be a major contribution to the solution of this problem. As stated by the senior author in another paper: "We are presenting a new era in disc syndrome management" [6, 7].

It is apparent that the technique described is most appropriate when there is one intervertebral disc involved in the pathologic process and that it is accessible to percutaneous puncture and that it is associated with bulging of the disc, but without actual rupture of the annulus to permit movement of the extruded fragment to a location that would not permit safe extraction of the fragment.

At the present time we are confining our recommendation for this type of percutaneous surgery to younger individuals without the complication of osteophytic overgrowth of the disc space and to individuals who can tolerate a procedure of one to one and a half hours under local anesthesia with supporting sedation, but without the need for general anesthesia.

Technique

1) Preparation of patient: The patient is told that this is a new technique; that due to technical difficulties, he or she may need the conventional operation, more often if the rupture is at the level of L 5–S 1.

[1] California Orthopedic Medical Clinic, Orthopedic Hospital, University of Southern California, Los Angeles, CA 90048, USA

Percutaneous Lumbar Discectomy
Ed. by H. M. Mayer and M. Brock

2) Anesthesia: The procedure is done under local anesthesia. The patient is better awake in order to inform the surgeon if the needle should strike a nerve root. This cooperation makes the procedure safer with respect to damage of the nerve root.

The presence of an anesthesiologist is valuable and recommended.

Facilities

a) C-arm image intensifier with double recorded screen is necessary for this technique.
b) Nucleotome, which consists of an 18 gauge guide pin, a dilator tube, a trephine, and the nucleotome probe. All are provided in a sterile disposable tray.

The nucleotome has a mobile probe that may pass the nucleus pulposus when it is used. The tip of the nucleotome is blunt to insure safe use. Inside the mechanism is a trephine, used in conjunction with the nucleotome to cut away the pieces of disc to be removed. An in-and-out flow of normal saline flushes these pieces away.

Position of the Patient

The patient should be positioned on his side over an x-ray transparent C-arm table (we prefer that the right side of the patient be up). A plastic bag of normal saline is put under the flank to make the spine straight or slightly convex-upward. The entire back is prepped and draped in the standard sterile manner. The C-arm is positioned over the lumbar spine. The midline of the spine is well-delineated. Comparison between the preoperative myelogram and MRI scan showing the level of interest is done, and the level to be operated on is specified by placing a small metal marker over the side of the patient.

Placement of the Guide Wire and the Actual Procedure

This is the single most important step of this procedure: First, the level of the involved disc is identified by putting a Steinmann pin over the side of the patient under guidance provided by the image intensifier.

Second, the skin, subcutaneous tissues and muscles 8 to 10 cm on the right side of the midline of the involved disc are infiltrated with 0.5% Marcaine. (Deep tissue near the disc is not anesthetized.)

Third, an 18-gauge guide wire 40 to 50 degrees from the vertical line and 8 to 10 cm from the midline is passed to hit the involved disc and enter into the nucleus pulposus under precise C-arm control. If one hits the nerve root, the patient will feel sharp pain radiating to his leg. Then the direction of the pin should be slightly changed. This is very important, and the purpose of doing the operation under local anesthesia is to avoid hitting the nerve root.

Fourth, roentgenograms (x-rays) are taken in the AP and lateral projections to confirm the position of the guide wire for documentation.

Fifth, a dilator tube is inserted over the guide wire and pushed until it rests against the annulus fibrosus. (One may feel the soft tissues of the annulus fibrosus as opposed to the harder bone tissue.)

Sixth, the inner tube of the dilator is replaced by a trephine, a similar tube with a cutting edge. When one uses this trephine, one feels the cutting of the annulus fibrosus when the tip of the trephine enters the nucleus pulposus.

Seventh, while holding the external tube firmly against the annulus fibrosus, the trephine is replaced with the nucleotome. The nucleotome is a double tube with double direction of fluid when in operation. The outer tube has a side-slide about 2 mm in size, while the inner tube has a sharp edge which runs against this side slide. The machine works with pressurized air and in-and-out flow, running during its function. The pieces come out of the nucleotome and will be transferred and collected in a tube for pathological tests.

Eighth, after rechecking that the nucleotome is in the center of the nucleus pulposus, the machine's function is started by use of a foot pedal switch connected to the special machine (Fig. 1).

Ninth, the operator must know when to start and when to stop the machine. The patient is awake during the entire procedure. As the machine starts to work, it takes 5 to 7 minutes until the air is evacuated and the first pieces of the disc start coming out. The machine must run continuously and be turned around until no

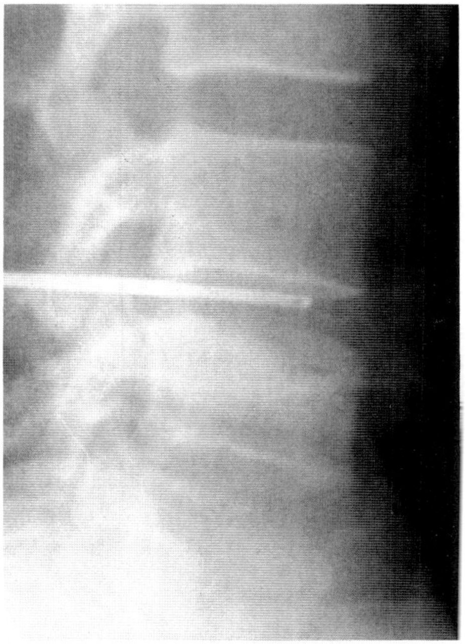

Fig. 1. Nucleotome probe placed in the intervertebral disc space in lateral x-ray projection

more pieces of disc are seen coming out. Normally this procedure takes 50 to 60 minutes for each level. One may check the probe of the nucleotome from time to time to be sure it isn't blocked.

Tenth, the operation is terminated, and the patient is kept under observation in the hospital for 24 hours. A mild antiinflammatory medication is prescribed for 10 to 14 days.

The patient may be discharged and sent home the following day. Hyperextension back exercises may start 7 days after the operation. The patient may return to light duty work in 1 to 7 days, and to regular duty work 4 to 6 weeks after surgery.

Results

Twenty-seven patients, aged 21 to 49, have been operated with this percutaneous technique. There were 22 male and five female patients. Three patients were eliminated because of shortage of follow-up. The patients came from physically active groups of our society; their occupations were a mixture of laborers in construction jobs, firemen and policemen.

All patients returned to their previous jobs at approximately six weeks postoperatively (Tables 1–4).

Table 1. Symptoms and signs

Criteria	Number of patients	%
Low back pain	24	96%
Leg or thigh pain	27	100%
Sensory deficit	27	100%
Motor weakness	20	60%

Table 2. Sex and jobs of 27 patients

Sex	Male	%	Female	%
Total	17	60	10	40
Light work, office work	6	20	5	20
Heavy work, laborer	11	40	5	20

Table 3. Age of patients

Age (years)	Male	%	Female	%	Total	%
10–20	0	0	0	0	0	0
20–30	6	20	4	10	10	30
30–40	6	20	3	15	9	35
40–50	5	20	3	15	8	35
over 50	0	0	0	0	0	0

Table 4. Results of surgery and return to work

Result of surgery	Number of patients	%
1. Patient satisfaction	26	94
2. Thigh or leg pain relieved	26	94
3. Back pain relieved	20	74
4. Return to previous job	25	92

Discussion

Post-laminectomy syndrome with epidural adhesions, spinal stenosis and spinal instability is well known to both neurosurgeons and orthopedic surgeons. A simple laminectomy similar to that done for human patients, was carried out on a group of (46) New Zealand white rabbits. Three to six months postoperatively, these animals began to exhibit neurological deficits, with kyphotic deformity of the lumbar spine. This experimental work led us to believe that the present standard techniques of laminectomy play a major role in producing postoperative complications and less than optimal results. It is in this respect that we welcome this newer technique of percutaneous discectomy which was first presented by Hijikata in 1975 [2–5]. We now have added our own experience in this matter and firmly believe that it is worthwhile to train and encourage our colleagues to treat their patients with this technique.

References

1. Dandy WE (1929) Loose cartilage from intervertebral disk simulating tumor of the spinal cord. Archieves of Surgery 19:660–672
2. Hijikata SA (1975) Percutane Nucleotomie – Neue Behandlung der Diskushernie. Journal of Toden Hospital 5:35
3. Kambin P, Gellmann H (1983) Percutaneous lateral discectomy of the lumbar spine. Clin Orth Rel Res 174:127–132
4. Morris J (1986) Percutaneous nucleotomy. Presented at the Advanced Symposium and Workshops on the Spine. Presented by the International College of Surgeons, Las Vegas/NV, March 1986
5. Onik G, Maroon JC (1987) Percutaneous automated discectomy: a new method for lumbar disc removal. J Neurosurgery 66:143–146
6. Rezaian SM (1988) New era in disc syndrome management, percutaneous discectomy. The Journal of Neurological and Orthopedic Medicine and Surgery 9/1
7. Rezaian SM et al. (1986) The result of simple laminectomy in rabbits. Presented at the Advanced Symposium and Workshops on the Spine, presented by the International College of Surgeons, Las Vegas/NV, March 1985

Experimental Approaches and Perspectives

The Possibilities of Percutaneous Lumbar Disc Surgery

J. A. N. SHEPPERD [1]

Introduction

The advent of percutaneous spinal surgery will produce no fundamental change to the principles of management in back pain and sciatica. Most symptoms from mechanical back pain will either resolve spontaneously, or would not justify surgery of any kind. Patients complain of pain and not abnormal x-rays or CT scans. The individual's perception and tolerance of pain is highly variable and needs most careful evaluation. Pain is probably caused by inflammation. This inflammation may result from mechanical or humoral factors. For example, it is known that an auto-immune response can occur when proteoglycans are released into contact with the immune system of the body. Also cervical and lumbar spines have been shown to generate high levels of leucotriene B4, which is one of the most potent inflammatory agents known. It is unlikely that symptoms based on humoral factors would respond to any conceivable form of surgery. Surgery for disc disorders has had a patchy track record and revision operations even more so.

In assessing pathology we have at our disposal clinical examination, x-rays, CT and MR for imaging abnormalities. The problem with these special investigations is that they may show irrelevant pathology or fail to demonstrate episodic conditions. They certainly fail to demonstrate dynamic events in a motion segment of the spine. Surrounded by humiliating uncertainty of diagnosis it is not surprising that results can disappoint, and there is little contention that a considerable number of patients believe themselves to be worse following a spinal procedure. Diagnostic accuracy may be improved by confirming that an apparently pathological structure causes the patient's symptoms when stimulated, where as when that same structure is eliminated the symptoms resolve. This principle has been applied in Hastings as the simplest form of percutaneous spinal disc procedure and is known as diagnostic spinal probing. The procedure precedes all percutaneous surgery.

[1] Hastings Orthopaedic Centre, Royal East Sussex Hospital Hastings, East Sussex TN34 1ER, England

Percutaneous Lumbar Discectomy
Ed. by H. M. Mayer and M. Brock

Diagnostic Probing

A specially designed radiolucent operating table adapter is used (Fig. 1). The patient is sedated by an anaesthetist experienced in the technique, titrating the conscious level to maintain a dialogue with the investigating surgeon. Using the posterolateral approach, a 1.5 mm dull-ended trocar and cannula is introduced on the side of the patient's symptoms. Stimulation is achieved by palpation pressure on the structure identified by x-ray. Also the trocar may be removed and a needle substituted by which fluid can be injected into facet joint capsule or disc to generate hydrostatic pressure. Contrast (Niopam) is used to outline the structure under consideration. Local anaesthetic is used to eliminate temporarily a suspected pain source. This is either by 2% lignocaine for an instant response, or 0.75% Marcaine for a sustained anaesthesia. A methodical probing routine is undertaken including the facet joint, the subfacet perinerve root region, the disc

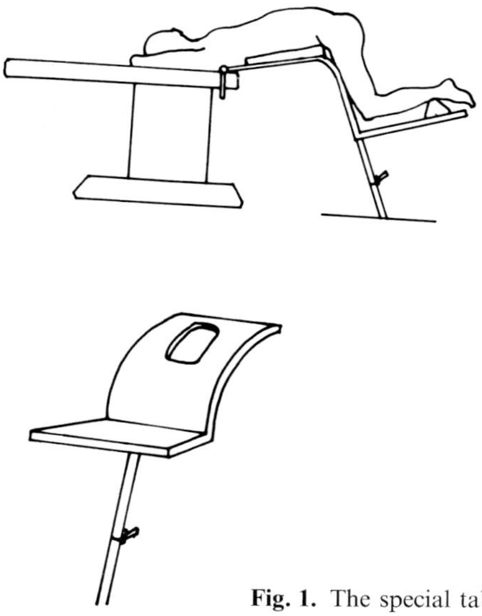

Fig. 1. The special table attachment used for percutaneous procedures

Table 1a, b. Results of spinal probing in 154 patients. **a** Pain source. **b** Sciatica, back pain and degenerative change

	a			b	
a	Facet joint alone	29	**b**	Prolapsed disc, symptoms of sciatica, confirmed triad	74
	Disc annulus alone	53		Back pain, segment, triad confirmed	31
	Facet and disc	45		Degenerate change, triad confirmed, 1 segment	22
	Diffuse pain, no diagnosis	27		No definite diagnosis	27
		154			154

periphery and lateral expansion of the longitudinal ligament and also a discogram. If this investigation suggests that a structure other than a suspect disc is accounting for symptoms, the structure is instilled with Marcaine and a local corticosteroid and the effect carefully evaluated on returning to the ward. Only if the diagnosis of a suspected disc protrusion is confirmed do we then proceed at the same time to percutaneous access and disc surgery.

We have now undertaken 900 spinal probes and an analysis of the procedure in 154 patients is included in Table 1.

Percutaneous Access

A needle with removable boss is placed through the probing cannula into the disc. The boss and cannula are then removed so that the needle acts as a guide wire. A series of coaxial tubes may be installed sequentially over the guide wire. The leading edge of the tubes is bevelled over a 2.5 mm length, to minimise trauma to the exiting nerve root or vessels. The bevel should be no greater. Cadaver studies have indicated that a tube up to 1 cm outside diameter can be used without any likelihood of nerve root damage provided the initial position of the needle is satisfactory. Discectomy is undertaken with a 3 or 4 mm tube, depending on the size of disc and objectives, and fusion procedures have been undertaken with the larger tubes.

Discectomy

Total discectomy would leave raw end plates, total loss of space and interbody fusion. This procedure is, of course, never done and discetomy by any conventional method is only partial. Using the percutaneous method the following options exist:

1) Removal of thin nucleus material from the disc centre. This may achieve reduction in intradiscal pressure both by the nucleotomy and reduction of proteoglycan-laden bulk. These factors may set the scene for healing of a disc herniation. This type of technique has been undertaken most widely using the automated Nucleotome, although other methods appear equally good. Satisfactory results could be expected within careful patient selection limits, and minimal reduction of disc height may obviate subsequent lateral recess entrapment.
2) In order to remove more bulky disc fragments, wider-bore instruments are required. Loose internal free fragments with a high collagen content are frequently found. When such free fragments contribute to disc instability and consequent symptoms, they are generally found in the posterior disc. Forward acting rongeurs by conventional or percutaneous methods may leave such material behind. By removal of only anterior material a wedge effect may be created which could increase retropulsion of the free fragment. To overcome this difficulty we

Fig. 2. Retroacting rongeurs, used for removing posterior disc material

Table 2. Results of nucleectomy and posterior discectomy in 68 patients (minimum follow-up six months)

	Nucleectomy (31)	Posterior discectomy (37)	Total (68)
Excellent	8 (26%)	11 (31%)	19 (27%)
Good	13 (42%)	19 (51%)	32 (47%)
Fair	5 (11%)	5 (12%)	10 (14%)
Open operation for failure	5 (11%)	2 (6%)	7 (10%)

Excellent = symptom-free; Good = very much better but minimal symptoms persisting; Fair = unimproved.

Table 3. Speed of recovery in 68 patients

	Nucleectomy (31)	Posterior discectomy (37)	Total (68)
Discharged within 24 hours	31	37	68 (100%)
In regular employment	18	30	48 (67%)
Return to work by 2 weeks	7	15	22 (45%)
Return to work by 6 weeks	12	26	38 (78%)

have introduced backward-acting rongeurs (Fig. 2). Negative pressure is created by a suction device that fits over the introduction tube, the intention being to encourage disc material towards a rongeur. Our results over a four year period are presented in Tables 2 and 3. It is possible that patients with leser pathology are more perceptive of the symptoms that they experience and if this is so it could explain apparently less satisfactory results following nucleus decompression rather than posterior discectomy. We believe that convincing posterolateral herniation in the absence of sequestration is better managed by forward- and backward-acting rongeurs when greater quantities of material are obtained. In judging the volume of material removed by any form of discectomy, due allowance must be made for the nucleus material to absorb water and, therefore swell the apparent volume.

3) Sequestrated fragments and lateral recess entrapment are unlikely to respond to intradiscal decompression, and where these are suspected we undertake an open procedure using a microdiscectomy method on the same table adaptor.

Spinal Fusion

Employing larger tubes (1 cm outside diameter) we have undertaken a series of distraction interbody fusions. The objective is to restore disc height, and thereby the lateral recess. The indication for fusion is back pain which is resolved temporarily by anaesthetisation of the segment to be fused (using the spinal probing technique described above). An assessment of potential percutaneous access is made at the same time but the definitive fusion procedure has been done under general anaesthetic.

A tapered broach is used to create an adequate access tunnel, before using the coaxial tubes in the conventional manner. Homograft bone has been employed, gas-sterilized on the lines of Cloward's recommendation.

Thorough disc clearance can be undertaken with bilateral placement of the larger tubes, and a small ring curette removes end plate cartilage. The introduction of an endoscope confirms adequate preparation of the graft bed. Bilateral dowel grafts are supplemented by piecemeal graft infill (Fig. 3).

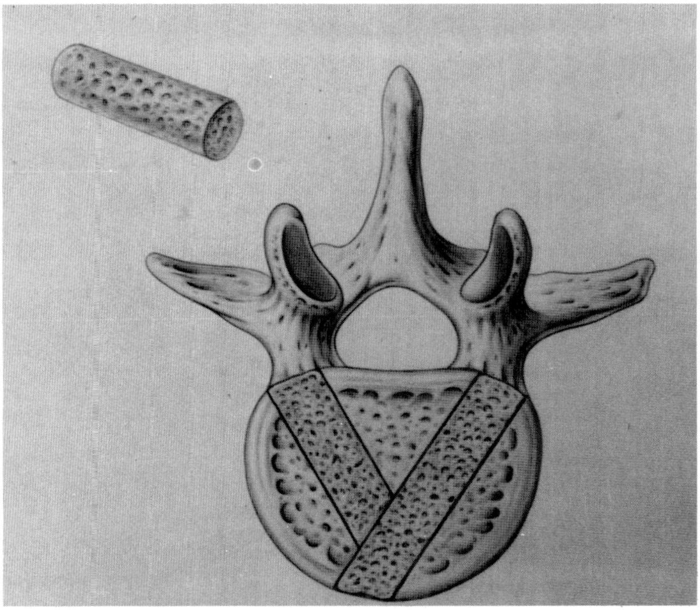

Fig. 3. Percutaneous fusion has been done with bilateral graft placement using homograft dowels and piecemeal infill

Table 4. Results (percutaneous fusion, 15 patients)

Satisfactory	8
Radiologically fused	6

The results of this procedure are given in Table 4. Because of the disappointing results we have abandoned this technique. At the present time we are developing the percutaneous method further. We believe that failure of fusion may be reduced by simultaneous anterior and posterior stabilisation, and that effective restoration of disc height requires an implant.

Percutaneous Endoscopic Laser Discectomy – Experimental Results

H. M. MAYER [1], M. BROCK [1], E. STEIN [2], and G. MÜLLER [2]

Introduction

The use of laser as a "surgical tool" has been widely accepted in medicine [1, 8, 9]. Laser is superior to mechanical instruments, especially in procedures which benefit from a no-touch technique, such as ablation, cutting or coagulation. The advantage of negligible trauma to structures surrounding the operating field is of utmost importance in neurosurgery. Thus, the use of laser has definitely improved the removal of brain tumors in critical locations [3, 5, 6, 9, 10]. Moreover, laser technology has led to a dramatic progress in endoscopic interventions. The higher flexibility achieved by the use of flexible quartz fibers permits the removal of normal or pathological tissue from the pulmonary or gastrointestinal tract [13].

The percutaneous treatment of lumbar disc herniations (percutaneous discectomy/nucleectomy) opens a new field for laser application [11].

The Use of Laser in Percutaneous Lumbar Discectomy (PLD)

The aim of PLD is the selective removal of non-sequestrated nucleus pulposus material under direct visual control. This selective nucleectomy leads to a decompression of the affected spinal nerve. The use of endoscopic techniques (discoscopy) is necessary [11, 14] (Fig. 1). To reach the most dorsal part of the disc, the instruments must be designed so as to fulfill the requirements for the posterolateral approach (Fig. 2) and must, in addition, display sufficient flexibility.

Solutions Without Laser

To remove nucleus material from the target regions, angled and flexible forceps are used. Moreover, shaver and cutter systems coupled to high-vacuum surgical suckers permit the removal of tissue from areas beyond the working range of the instruments (see page 107).

[1] Neurochirurgische Klinik, Klinikum Steglitz, Freie Universität Berlin, Hindenburgdamm 30, 1000 Berlin 45, FRG

[2] Lasermedizin-Zentrum Berlin GmbH, Krahmerstraße 6–10, 1000 Berlin 45, FRG

Percutaneous Lumbar Discectomy
Ed. by H. M. Mayer and M. Brock

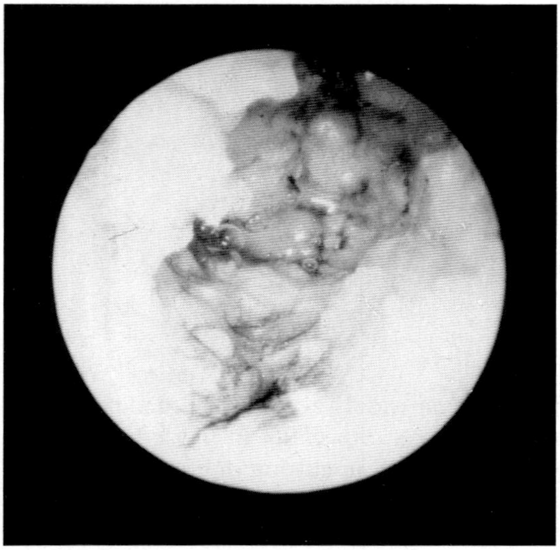

Fig. 1. Discoscopic view of a partially removed nucleus pulposus

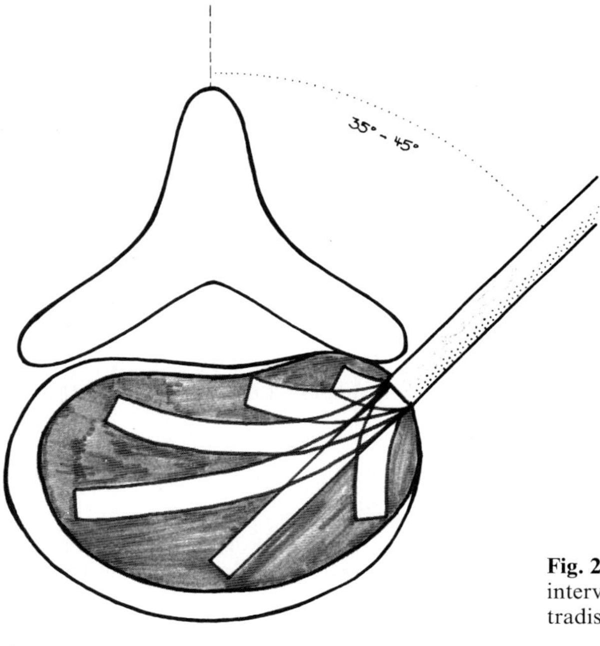

Fig. 2. Percutaneous approach to the intervertebral space and required intradiscal working range

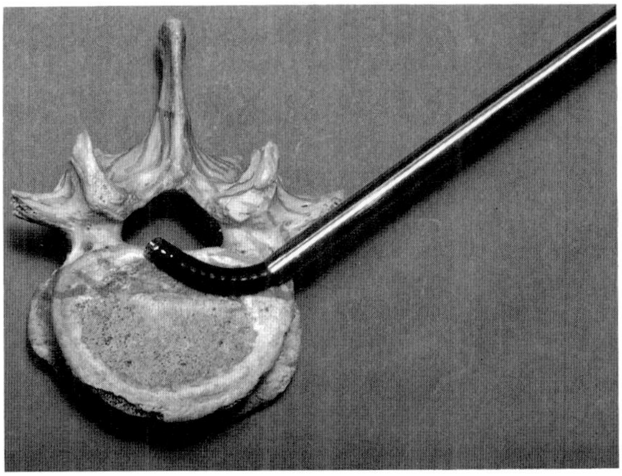

Fig. 3. Flexible endoscope introduced into the intervertebral space through PLD working cannula

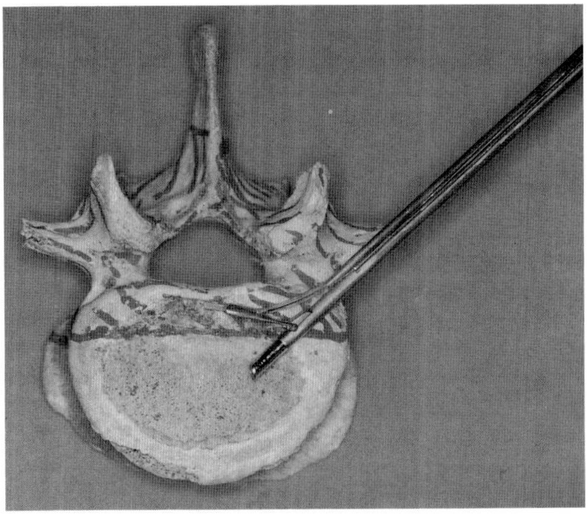

Fig. 4. Rigid endoscope with Albaran device to direct a quartz fiber

Solutions with Laser

The effective use of forceps or cutter systems under permanent visual control requires a second percutaneous approach from the opposite side for the endoscope [14]. This poses no technical problem but prolongs the surgical procedure and might increase the risk of disc-space infection. As opposed to this, selective vaporization or photodisruption of parts of the nucleus pulposus should be possible through one single flexible (Fig. 3) or rigid angled endoscope (Fig. 4) coupled to a laser source. The removal of nucleus pulposus would thus be possible under visual control via a single approach. The intradiscal steps of the procedure would be atraumatic as compared to the use of forceps, provided the hazards of the laser technique are mastered.

What Kind of Laser?

To be most effective in percutaneous discectomy, the laser light should have a wavelength of high absorption, low reflection, low scattering, and low transmission within the nucleus pulposus tissue.

Potential hazards arising from temperature effects or from a direct lesion to the surrounding structures should be controllable. Laser parameters should allow the vaporization of a predictable volume of tissue.

Experimental Studies

A series of experiments was performed to find the "ideal" laser for the removal of nucleus pulposus tissue.

Based on the clinical experience with Neodymium: YAG-laser (1318 nm) and the physical properties of the Erbium: YAG-laser (2940 nm), experiments were carried out first with these two types of laser. Since both are effective in either coagulation or carbonization and vaporization of a considerable amount of tissue in an acceptable time, the studies were restricted to the transmission of laser energy through the disc.

Material and Methods

The experiments were carried out on ten fresh human lumbar disc specimens (levels L 3/4 and L 4/5) obtained at autopsy. The age of the deceased was between 46 and 59 years. The lumbar discs showed only moderate macroscopic signs of degeneration.

Experiments were carried out at room temperature. The lasers investigated were a Nd:YAG laser (1318 nm, MBB, München, FRG) and an Erbium:YAG laser (2940 nm MBB, München, FRG). The energy was applied through a 600-μm quartz fiber (Nd:YAG laser) or through a rigid optical system (Erbium:YAG laser). The Nd:YAG-laser was used in the continuous wave mode, the Erbium:YAG-lasers in a pulsed mode with a frequency of 14 Hz.

Transmission (%) through annulus fibrosus and nucleus pulposus were calculated [12]. The measurements were performed using a disc calorimeter (Rofin-Sinar Laser Powermeter, Ophir Optics Ltd., Jerusalem, Israel). The sensor diameter was 20 mm. The laser was installed at a distance of 12 mm above the sensor, and an initial reading (E0) was obtained with only air between the laser and the sensor. The energy range used was 11.43–96 J (Nd:YAG 1318) and 0.39–45.7 J (Erbium:YAG 2940). The exposure times were 1, 2, 3, 4 and 5 s. Each measurement was repeated three times, the arithmetic average was used for calculations. Following the initial readings, a tissue block (d = 10 mm) of either annulus fibrosus or nucleus pulposus was placed between the sensor and the laser source, and the measurements were repeated under otherwise identical conditions. The position of the tissue block was changed following each application to avoid double exposition. The percentage transmission (%) was calculated. Reflection and scattering of Laser energy were not taken into account.

Results

Neodymium:YAG 1318 mm
The applied energy (E0) is given in Table 1.

Nucleus pulposus:
Carbonization of nucleus pulposus started at 59.64 J. The transmitted energy (E) ranged between 0.79 and 9.1 J. The E0 value at the "carbonization threshold" (C) was 59.64 J and the transmission reached 9.4%. It ranged between 3.9 and 10.5%; however, values beyond the carbonization threshold are not corrected for the tissue thickness, which changes with carbonization (Table 2 and Fig. 5).

Annulus fibrosus:
No visible carbonization or vaporization could be observed with the energies used. The transmission ranged from 4.78 to 9.11% (Table 3 and Fig. 6).

Table 1. Initial energy (E_0) at the distal end of a 600 μm quartz fiber (Nd:YAG 1318 nm)

T (s)	E_0 (J)	
	1	2
1	11.43	19.9
2	24.58	39.76
3	37.2	59.64 C
4	46.48	79.4
5	62.35	96

Table 2. Nd:YAG 1318 nm, energy transmission through a 10 mm tissue block of nucleus pulposus

T (s)	Transmission (%)	
	1	2
1	10.5	3.9
2	9	4
3	8.6	9.4 C
4	9	8.3
5	–	9.4
$\bar{X}$	9.3	7.1
sx	0.7	2.7

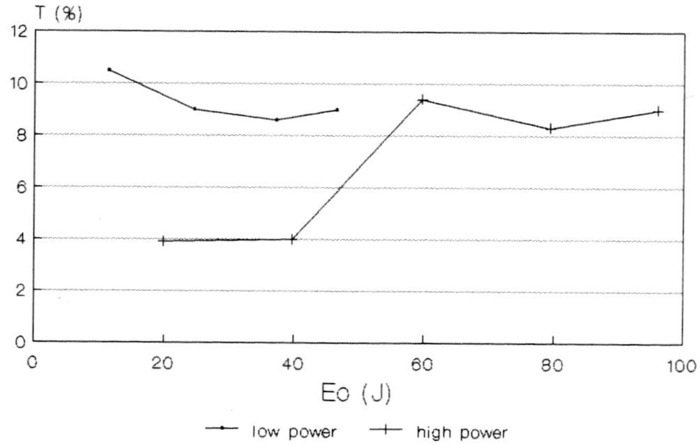

Fig. 5. Transmission (%) of Nd:YAG 1318-energy applied to a 10 mm tissue block of human nucleus pulposus

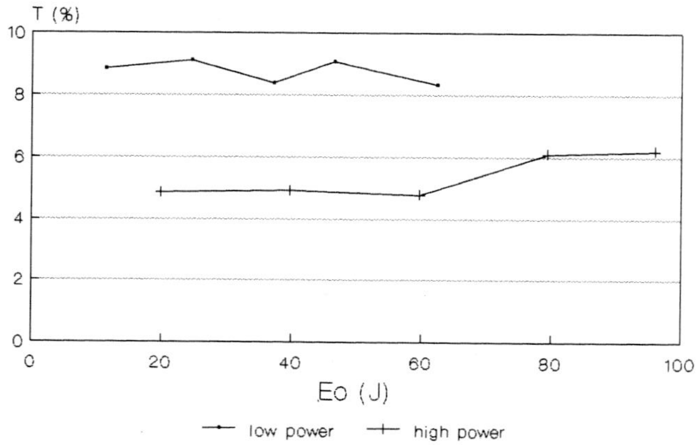

Fig. 6. Transmission (%) of Nd:YAG 1318-energy applied to a 10 mm tissue block of annulus fibrosus

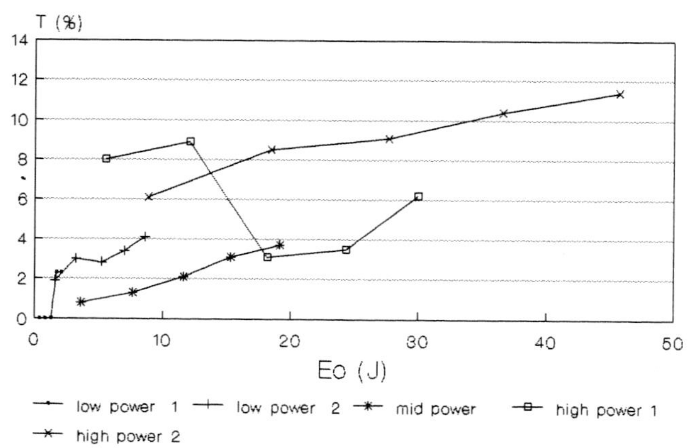

Fig. 7. Transmission (%) of Erb:YAG 2940-energy applied to a 10 mm tissue block of human nucleus pulposus

Table 3. Nd:YAG 1318 nm, energy transmission through a 10 mm tissue block of annulus fibrosus

T (s)	Transmission (%)	
	1	2
1	8.84	4.87
2	9.11	4.93
3	8.39	4.78
4	9.08	6.1
5	8.34	6.2
$\bar{X}$	8.75	5.38
sx	0.33	0.63

Table 4. Initial energy (E_0) Erb:YAG 2940 nm

T (s)	E_0 (J)				
	1	2	3	4	5
1	0.39	1.59	3.65	5.53	8.86
2	0.82	3.28 V	7.68	12.08	18.42
3	1.29	5.28	11.61	18.15	27.66
4	1.72	7	15.32	24.32	36.56
5	2.15	8.6	19.15	29.95	45.7

Table 5. Erb:YAG 2940 nm, energy transmission through a 10 mm tissue block of nucleus pulposus

T (s)	Transmission (%)				
	1	2	3	4	5
1	0	1.9	0.8	8	6.1
2	0	3 V	1.3	8.9	8.5
3	0	2.8	2.1	3.1	9.1
4	2.3	3.4	3.1	3.5	10.4
5	2.3	4.1	3.7	6.2	11.4
$\bar{X}$	0.9	3	2.2	5.9	9.1
sx	1.1	0.7	1.1	2.3	1.8

Erbium:YAG 2940 nm
The energies applied are listed in Table 4.

Nucleus pulposus:
Visible vaporization of nucleus pulposus started at an applied energy level of 3.28 J. The transmitted energy (E) ranged between 0 and 5.2 J. The E0 value at the "vaporization threshold" was 0.1 and 3% for transmission. The transmission ranged between 0 and 11.4% (Table 5 and Fig. 7).

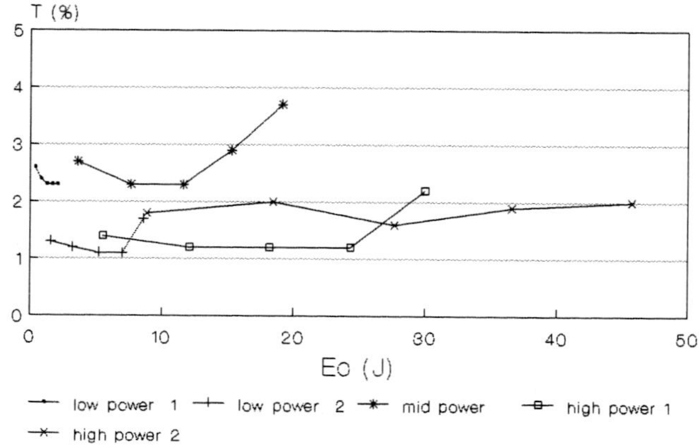

Fig. 8. Transmission (%) of Erb:YAG 2940-energy applied to a 10 mm tissue block of human annulus fibrosus

Table 6. Erb:YAG 2940 nm, energy transmission through a 10 mm tissue block of annulus fibrosus

T (s)	Transmission (%)				
	1	2	3	4	5
1	2.6	1.3	2.7 V	1.4	1.8
2	2.4	1.2	2.3	1.2	2
3	2.3	1.1	2.3	1.2	1.6
4	2.3	1.1	2.9	1.2	1.9
5	2.3	1.7	3.7	2.2	2
$\bar{X}$	2.4	1.3	2.8	1.4	1.9
SX	0.1	0.2	0.5	0.4	0.1

Annulus fibrosus:
Vaporization started at an applied energy level of 3.65. Transmitted energy ranged between 0.01 and 0.9. The (E)-value at the "vaporization threshold" was 0.1 J and 2.7% for transmission. The transmission ranged between 1.1 and 3.7% (Table 6 and Fig. 8).

Conclusions

The effect of laser light on biological tissues is determined by the laser wavelength, application power, application time, physical properties of the laser beam, and by the physical properties of the tissue [1, 7, 8]. The absorption spectra of human nucleus pulposus and annulus fibrosus did not show any tissue-specific peak. Most of the energy is absorbed by water at wavelengths in the far infrared range [12]. Taking these observations into account, one can predict a low vaporization effect

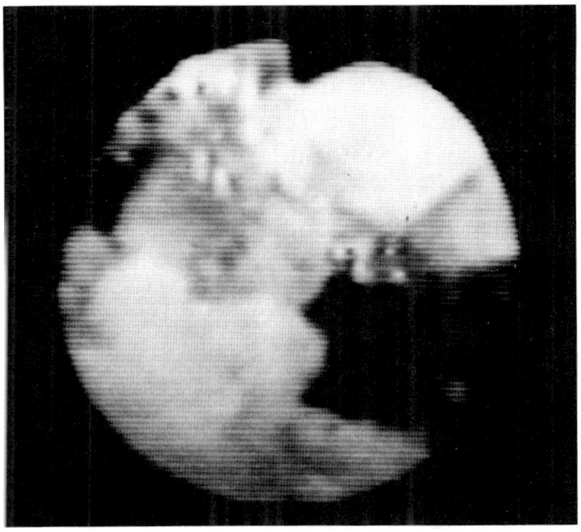

Fig. 9. Experimental endoscopic laser discectomy using a flexible endoscope. The quartz fiber is visible (at 3 o'clock) at the distal end of the endoscope introduced into the intervertebral space

of Neodymium:YAG lasers at wavelengths of 1060 and 1320 nm. This has already been demonstrated experimentally and in preliminary clinical studies [2, 3, 15]. The mechanism of tissue removal by Neodymium:YAG lasers is based on the temperature effect. The application in the lumbar disc space with or without endoscopic control bears the risk of heat damage not only to the surrounding structures but also to the vertebral end-plates, which are most important in the homeostasis of the lumbar disc. Thermographic measurements during disc carbonization with Nd:YAG 1064 nm cw lasers demonstrated perifocal temperature rises of more than 60° C near to the endplates, but failed to demonstrate any dangerous temperature effect in the periphery of the disc. This hazard can be minimized using a pulsed mode laser application [12]. Our experiments demonstrate that, besides a rather limited removal of tissue by the Nd:YAG 1318 laser, the transmission of energy through nucleus pulposus and annulus fibrosus is 10.5 and 9.1% respectively. Although a maximum of 9.1% of the energy is transmitted through 10 mm of annulus fibrosus, no carbonization effect could be demonstrated. The effect of transmitted energy should not be underestimated since it might cause tissue damage to sensitive structures outside the disc space. A similar effect was observed in the neurosurgical removal of falx meningiomas with a Neodymium:YAG laser, where a subsequent necrosis of cerebral cortex of the opposite hemisphere occurred due to energy transmitted through the falx cerebri [4]. Thus, the procedure should always be controlled endoscopically (Fig. 9).

Erbium:YAG laser energy has a high absorption in water. Since even degenerated lumbar discs contain about 75% of water, a good effect of this type of laser could be predicted. It was shown that nucleus pulposus as well as annulus fibrosus can be vaporized with low energy and low temperature effects. The transmitted energy is low and does not exceed 3% at the vaporization threshold.

Even if one considers that transmission values beyond the vaporization threshold are not corrected for the different tissue thicknesses, reflection and scattering, they do not exceed 3.7% for the annulus fibrosus and 11.4% for the nucleus pulposus.

In conclusion, the Nd:YAG 1318 laser is useful for coagulation and carbonization of nucleus pulposus. High energies are necessary for effective removal of the nucleus; the transmitted energy exceeds 10%. It should be applied only with endoscopic control. Temperature effects can be minimized using a pulsed application mode. Flexible endoscopes are available and allow endoscopic photonucleolysis. Selective vaporization of the nucleus might, however, be accompanied by temperature effects mainly in the endplates.

The Erbium-YAG 2940 laser ensures an effective and selective nucleectomy. Temperature effects as well as transmission of energy through the tissue are low. Endoscopic application, however, still depends on the development of more adequate flexible fibers or rigid optical systems – technical problems to be solved in the near future.

It is considered that, eventually, percutaneous endoscopic discectomy will permit selective ("color-steered") removal of disc material at any point of the intervertebral space in an efficient and atraumatic way. A prerequisite, however, is the development of adequate instrumentation.

References

1. Apfelberg D (ed) (1981) Evaluation and installation of surgical laser-systems. Springer, Berlin Heidelberg New York
2. Ascher PW (1986) Application of the laser in neurosurgery. Laser in Med and Surg 2: 91–97
3. Ascher WP (1988) Laser in der Neurochirurgie. In: Walter W, Krenkel W (Hrsg) Jahrbuch der Neurochirurgie 1988, pp 101–119
4. Ascher WP, personal communication
5. Auer LM Ascher PW, Holzer P (1987) Laser-assisted neurosurgical endoscopy. Laser in Med and Surg 3: 114–119
6. Beck OJ, Frank F (1984) Nd:YAG Laser in der Neurochirurgie. MMW 126(5): 109–113
7. Berlien HP, Müller G (eds) (1988) Angewandte Lasermedizin. ECO-MED-Verlag, Landsberg
8. Frank F (1987) Der Laser in Chirurgie und Endoskopie. Dt Aerzteblatt 84(47): 2238–2343
9. Frank F, Beck OJ, Keiditsch JL et al. (1987) Investigations under neurosurgical aspects with the 1,32 μm Nd:YAG laser. Laser in Med and Surg 3: 40–44
10. Kelly PJ, Kall BA, Goerss S, Earnest F (1986) Computer-assisted stereotaxic laser resection of intra-axial brain neoplasms. J Neurosurg 64: 427–439
11. Mayer HM, Brock M (1988) Die perkutane Diskektomie. Dt Aerzteblatt 85: 853–858
12. Mayer HM et al., in preparation
13. Ossoff RH, Duncavage JA (1987) Past, present and future usage of lasers in otolaryngology – head and neck surgery. In: Apfelberg DB (ed) Evaluation and installation of surgical laser systems, pp 127–149
14. Schreiber A, Suezawa Y (1986) Transdiscoscopic percutaneous nucleotomy in disk herniation. Orth Rev 15: 75–78
15. Wharen RE, Anderson RE, Scheithauer B, Sundt TM (1984) The Nd:YAG laser in neurosurgery. Part 1: Laboratory investigations: dose-related biological response of neural tissue. J Neurosurg 60: 531–539

Percutaneous Intradiscal Laser Discectomy

T. YONEZAWA [1], S. TANAKA [1], H. WATANABE [1], T. ONOMURA [1], and K. ATSUMI [2]

Introduction

Recently percutaneous discectomy, such as chemonucleolysis with chymopapain [1] and percutaneous nucleotomy with punch [2] or nucleotome, has been developed extensively in Europe and America to provide an alternative to surgery in the treatment of lumbar disc herniation. But percutaneous nucleotomy, as mentioned above, has not been used in our daily therapy because of the limitation of indication, complications and technical problems. The experimental study of percutaneous intradiscal laser discectomy (PILD) has been tried to provide an alternative to percutaneous discectomies which are currently applied. The protocol of our study was composed of five parts. The five parts were as follows: 1) The optimum condition was obtained to vaporizes nucleus pulposus with Nd:YAG laser using sacrificed rabbit and goat lumbar discs. 2) The intradiscal changes in the time course were observed by microscopic evaluation using rabbit lumbar discs. 3) The relationship between intradiscal pressure (IDP) and vertical load in the time course were compared between irradiated discs, normal discs and control discs which were operated by curette. 4) Fibers and needles were developed to diminish heat damage. 5) Preliminary in vivo trial of PILD was performed in anesthetized young goats under X-ray guidance prior to the application for human cases.

Materials and Methods

Materials: Rabbit and goat lumbar discs were used for in vitro and in vivo experiments.

Instruments: Nd:YAG laser (1.06 micron wave length, made by Osada Electric, Co.), spinal needles and new type double lumen needles coated with Teflon, which have a connector for aspiration and quartz fibers (400, 300 and 200 micron in diameter), were used.

[1] Department of Orthopedics, Osaka Medical College, Daigaku-cyou, Takatsuki, Osaka, Japan
[2] Institute of Medical Electronics, Faculty of Medicine, University of Tokyo, Tokyo, Japan

Percutaneous Lumbar Discectomy
Ed. by H.M. Mayer and M. Brock

Methods: The tip of the needle was fixed at the center of the vertebral disc under direct visual or X-ray control and a fiber was inserted near the tip of the needle. Then the tissue was irradiated with Nd:YAG laser. After irradiation, the animals were sacrificed for each study.

1) Determination of the optimum conditions to vaporize nucleus pulposus using sacrificed rabbit and goat lumbar discs: 400 micron quartz fiber and 18 G and 20 G spinal needles were used. The duration of laser irradiation was 0.3 to 0.5 seconds with a power of 30, 40 and 50 watts alternating with 1.5 to 2.0 seconds pauses. The repetition times were 10 to 50 times. Tissues were stained with H.E., H.E. elastica and toluidine blue.

2) Determination of the histological changes in the time course after laser irradiation: 8 rabbits anesthetized with pentobarbital were irradiated under direct visual control: 400 micron quartz fiber and 20 G spinal needle were used. The duration of laser irradiation was 0.3 seconds with a power of 30 watts and an interval of 1.5 to 2.0 seconds. The pulse was repeated 25 to 30 times.

3) Determination of the intradiscal pressure in the time course after laser irradiation: 5 anesthetized rabbits which were irradiated with laser under the same condition as mentioned above and 2 rabbits which were operated by curette as control were sacrificed. Discs were cut down at each segment and the intradiscal pressures were measured with compression tester, load cell and a pressure transducer [4].

4) In the experiments 1–3, the heat damages of surrounding tissues, seem to be the major technical problem. Then new needles and fibers were developed according to the evaluation of thermal distribution with infra-red thermography and thermocouples. Thermographical image had been recorded 25 slices of image per 1 second on a screen. The temperature was measured at 4 points by thermocouples.

5) Preliminary in vivo trial of PILD to kids anesthetized with GOF or pentobarbital under X-ray guidance: A double lumen needle with 19 G or 18 G outer needle, 23 G inner needle and 200 micron bare quartz fiber was used (Fig. 1). The duration of laser irradiation was 0.3 seconds with a power of 15 watts and an interval of 1.5 to 2.0 seconds. The pulse was repeated for 50 to 60 times with 65 to 70 cmHg aspiration.

Results

1) The optimum laser irradiating conditions without damages of surrounding tissues are as follows (Fig. 2):

	Power (watts)	Duration of laser irradiation	Interval	Repetition (times)
Rabbit:	30	0.4 s	1.5 to 2.0 s	25 to 30
Goat:	40	0.4 s	1.5 to 2.0 s	40 to 45

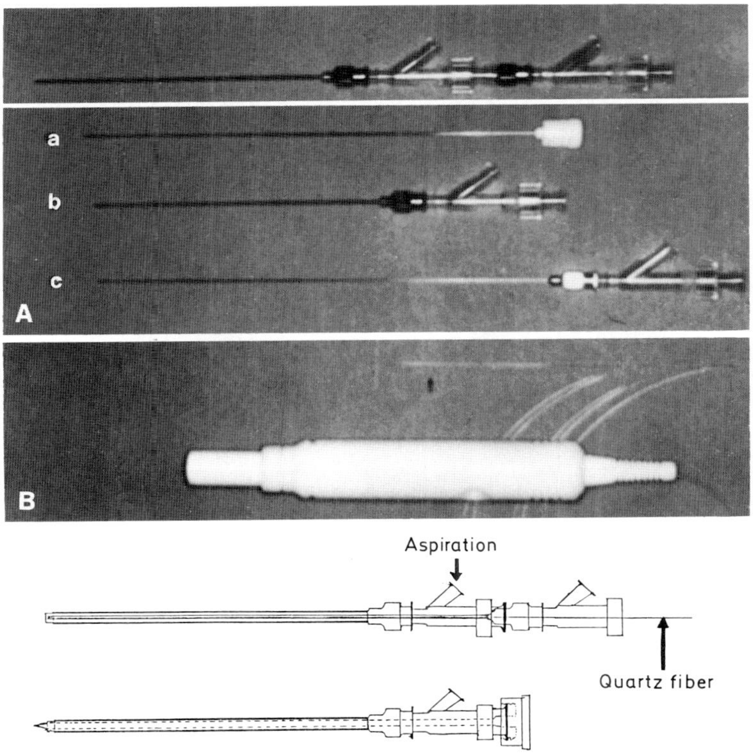

Fig. 1 A, B. A new double lumen needle and 200 micron bare quartz fiber (disposable instruments). **A** A new double lumen needle. *a* insertion needle; *b*, *c* outer and inner needles. **B** A disposable type bare quartz fiber (200 micron in diameter)

Quartz fiber and needle were often destroyed with tissue burn back. At the moment of destruction, the distribution of high temperature, over 200 degrees centigrade as measured with thermography, was spread beyond annulus.

2) Histological findings after one day, 1 and 2 weeks revealed that the nucleus pulposus was vaporized and a cavity was made. Heat degeneration also occurred around the cavity. After 3 and 4 weeks, cartilaginous cells and fibrous tissues were beginning to proliferate. After 8 weeks, cartilaginous fibrous tissue nearly replaced cavity and lumbar spine had no instability (Fig. 3).

3) The IDP of vaporized discs and control discs operated with bone curette was 0 kg/cm^2 at 0 load, whereas in normal discs IDP was about 4 kg/cm^2. The vaporized disc IDP and operated disc IDP with bone curette elevated gently in proportion to the load ($Y = a\,X$, $a < 1$). On the other hand, the normal disc IDP elevated steeply ($Y = a\,X + 4$, $a > 1$) (Fig. 4).

4a) The results of thermal distribution using 200 micron diameter quartz fiber and 17 G and 21 G needles were as follows: The temperature at the center of

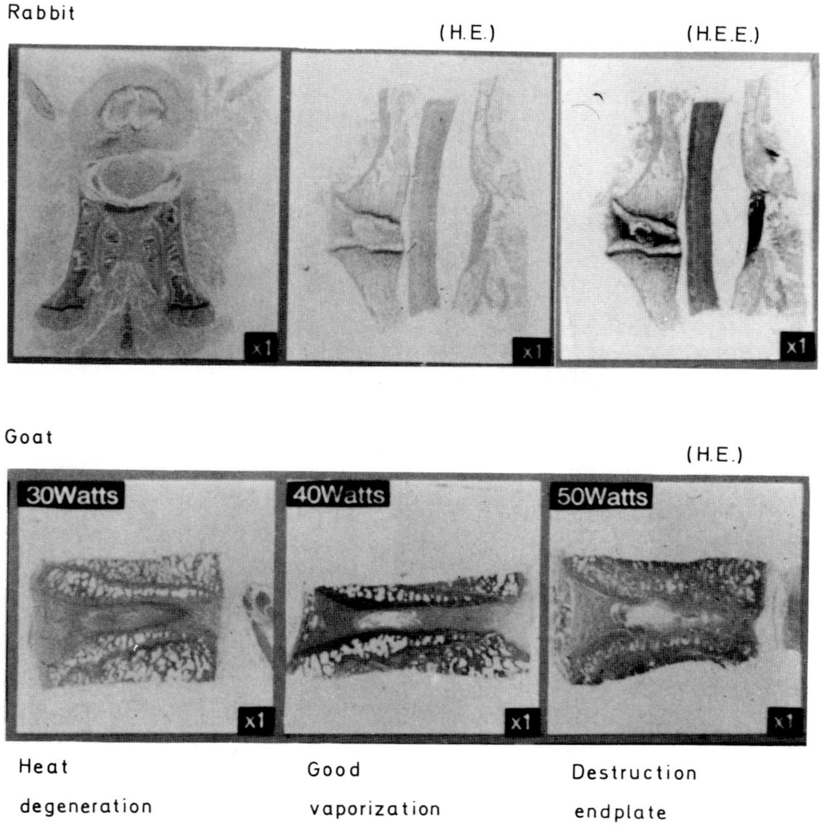

Fig. 2. Acute histological changes (immediately after irradiation). Irradiating conditions, such as power, duration, interval and pulse frequence were changed. Under optimum conditions, only nucleus pulposus was vaporized. H.E. and H.E. elastica stain

nucleus pulposus rose to about 190 degrees centigrade, while the temperature in annulus did not exceed 38 degrees centigrade. Destruction of the needle and quartz fiber did not occur within 60 repetitions.

4b) During the aspiration, the air temperatures at four points in the room did not exceed 30 degrees centigrade.

5) The procedure in goat lumbar discs is as follows (Fig. 5):

(1) A needle is inserted via a left lateral approach. The tip of the needle is set at the center of the nucleus pulposus under the aid of A-P and lateral X-ray view.

(2) Then discography is done to confirm the diagnosis and the position of the needle tip.

(3) Laser irradiation is performed about a few minutes. After laser irradiation, discography is done again to confirm the irradiating point and surrounding tissues condition.

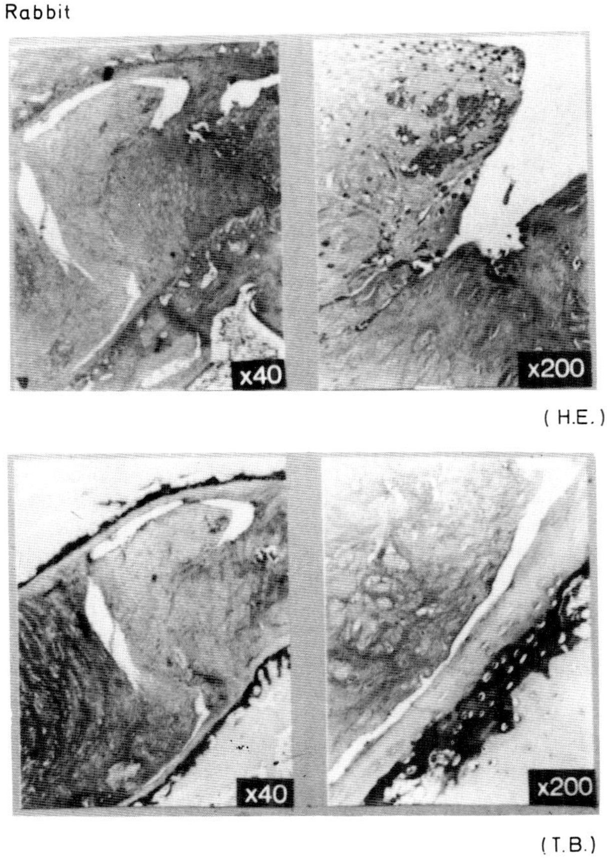

Fig. 3. Chronic histological changes (rabbit lumbar disc after 8 weeks). Cartilaginous cells and fibrous tissue are recognized obviously. H.E. and toluidine blue stain

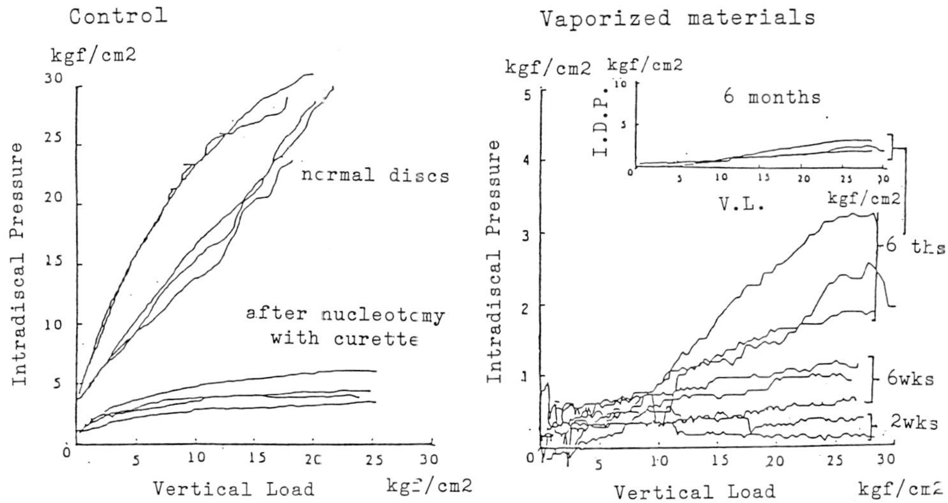

Fig. 4. The relationship between intradiscal pressure and vertical load. Normal disc curve: $Y = aX + 4$, $a > 1$. Vaporized disc and disc nucleotomized, with curette: $Y = aX + 0$, $a < 1$

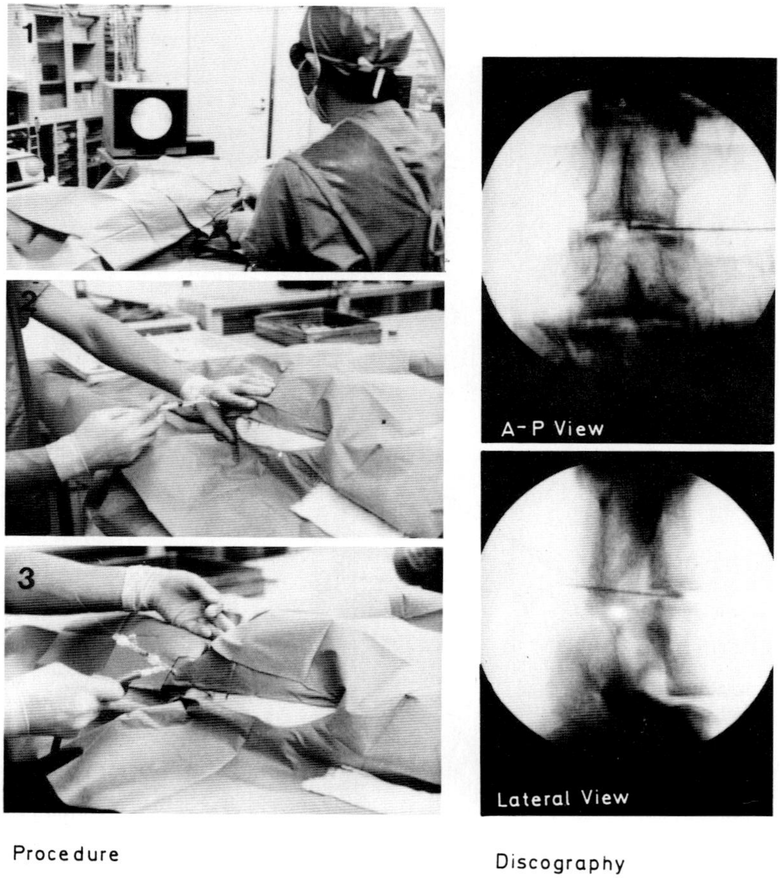

Fig. 5. Procedure of percutaneous intradiscal laser discectomy. The instruments consist of a new double needle, quartz fiber, radiopaque agents and eye-protecting glasses. *1.* Insertion of the needle through left lateral approach; *2.* discography through outer needle; *3.* laser irradiation. After the operation, discography is repeated

Discussion

It is well known from clinical and basic studies that the reduction of the IDP and stabilization of vertebra are effective in relieving sciatica caused by a herniated lumbar disc, such as the experimental studies of partial nucleotomy and fenestration by Hult and Olsson [3, 6], chemonucleolysis with chymopapain [8] and the clinical reports of anterior fusion [5]. The percutaneous discectomy cannot remove herniated mass. Chemonucleolysis and percutaneous nucleotomy have proved to be effective in many cases. However, the current methods of percutaneous discectomy have advantages and disadvantages. The procedure of chemonucleolysis is very easy and takes less operation time. However, complications

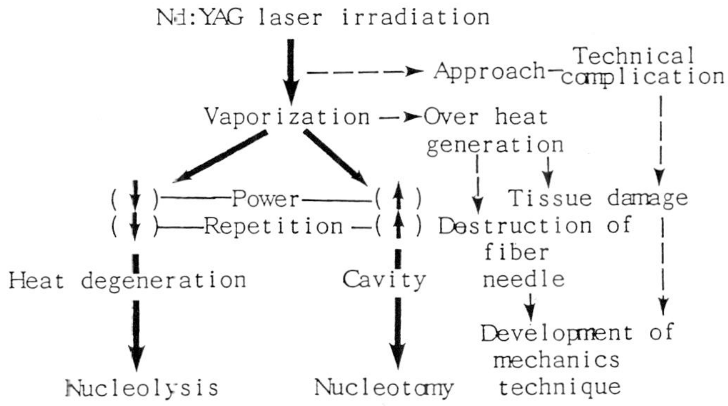

Fig. 6. Hypothesis of the effect of percutaneous intradiscal laser discectomy

such as anaphylactic shock, paraplegia, etc. occur in 1 to 3% as reported by Watts [9]. The incidence is very rare but should not be ignored. And chemonucleolysis has a limited effect in degenerated discs, because the amount of the substrate to be hydrolyzed by chymopapain is low. The diameter of the needles used in percutaneous nucleotomy by punch forceps is more than 3 mm, which may cause more technical problems and tissue damages than chemonucleolysis and PILD.

Though PILD is now in the experimental stage, results 1 and 2 showed that histological changes were the same as the changes following conventional nucleotomy reported by Hass in 1946 [1]. And result 3 meant almost the same effect of diminishing the IDP as that of percutaneous nucleotomy. From result 4, we are now able to use new instruments in in vivo experiments of PILD using anesthetized goats without many of the difficulties caused by insertion technique and temperature [7, 8].

If PILD may be used clinically, it has no fatal complications such as anaphylactic shock. Moreover, PILD has wider indication than chemonucleolysis, because the vaporization of matrix induce the same effect as that of nucleotomy even if the disc has degenerated by aging. Of course, if the disc, like a young person's disc, has not been degenerated, it is enough to vaporize tissue water at low power or with less repetition of laser irradiation (Fig. 6). And the diameter of the needle used in PILD is smaller than those used in percutaneous nucleotomy. It should cause less technical complications and take less operation time than percutaneous nucleotomy.

Conclusion

These experimental in vitro and in vivo studies using animals have shown that percutaneous intradiscal laser discectomy might have a wider indication and fewer complications than current methods of percutaneous discectomy. Moreover, this method is easy, safe, and takes only a few minutes of laser irradiation.

References

1. Haas SL (1949) Resection of intervertebral disc through the posterior approach. Arch Surg 59:1261–1264
2. Hijikata S (1979) Percutaneous nucleotomy. MOOK series of Orthopedics 11:246–265
3. Hult L (1950) Retroperitoneal disc fenestration on low back pain and sciatica. Acta Orthop Scand 20:342–348
4. Nachemson A (1981) Disc pressure measurements. Spine 6(1):93–97
5. Nakano N (1976) Youtuu no Rinshou (Clinic of Lumbago) 2nd ed. Nankou-dou, Tokyo, Japan, pp 173–217
6. Olsson SE (1950) Observation concerning disc fenestration in dog. Acta Orthop Scand 30:349–356
7. Smith L (1967) Treatment of lumbar intervertebral disc lesion by direct injection of chymopapain. J Bone Joint Surg 49(B):502–519
8. Takahashi K (1984) Biomechanical study on the effect of chymopapain to the intervertebral disk. Biomechanics of Orthopedics 6:7–11
9. Watts C (1977) Complications of chemonucleolysis for lumbar disc disease. Neurosurgery 1:2–5

Nucleus Pulposus Vaporization – Experimental Investigations on Use of Lasers on the Intervertebral Disc

W. E. Siebert and C. J. Wirth [1]

Introduction

Use of lasers is already widespread in extensive fields of surgical medicine, in particular owing to its great safety and exact controllability, but also because of the possibility of bringing high energy to the site of action with minimal instruments [16]. The idea of using a laser for treatment of a nonsequestrated intervertebral disc prolapse was logical because of the properties mentioned above. The search for a less invasive method of treatment which hardly burdens the patient for the often very painful protrusion, especially in the region of the lumbar spine, has become important not least in view of studies which criticize the effectiveness of chemonucleolysis [9, 11]. The fundamental idea of "nucleus pulposus vaporization" was to reduce by direct vaporization the optically very homogeneous properties of the nucleus pulposus, which differ substantially from the annulus fibrosus at least in healthy persons, and thus to attain decompression in the intervertebral disc concerned. At the same time, it was hoped that this technique would disturb the stability of the movement segments as little as possible owing to the small operation and the selective technique [2, 3, 6].

The word laser is an acronym from "light amplification by stimulated emission of radiation". The laser is thus essentially a light source with properties which occur in this combination only in the laser. These properties characterize the laser and obey the principles of optics.

The properties of a laser can only be dealt with briefly here. It is important that the radiation is strictly monochromatic, that it is coherent and that it is collimated.

Materials and Methods

Fundamental considerations in terms of our study objective and examination of the instruments for medical use available on the market [1, 5, 7, 8, 12, 14, 17], only left the CO_2 laser and the neodymium: YAG laser as feasible for our experiments on cadaver tissues.

[1] Orthopädische Klinik der Medizinischen Hochschule Hannover, Heimchenstraße 1–7, 3000 Hannover 61, FRG

Percutaneous Lumbar Discectomy
Ed. by H. M. Mayer and M. Brock

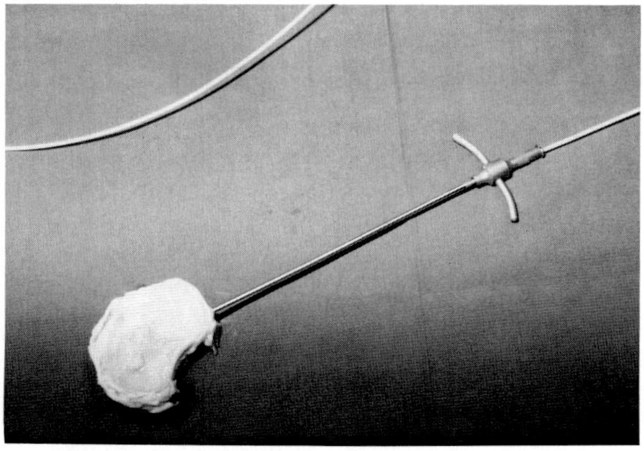

Fig. 1. Our original neodymium: YAG light conductor and the introduction needle in the preparation with still appreciable thickness and stiffness

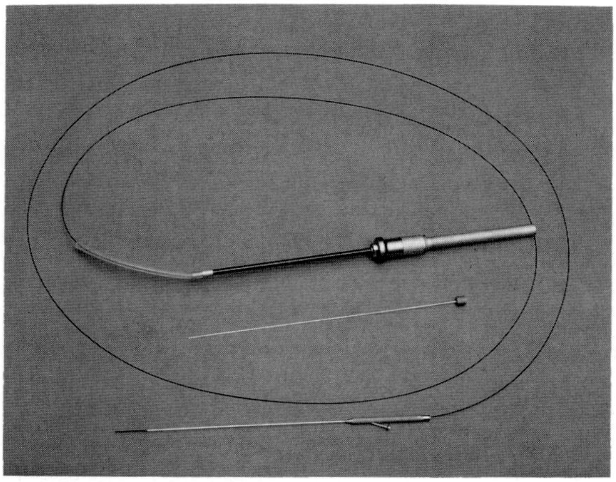

Fig. 2. The introduction instrument with 1 mm external diameter and the light conductor with a diameter of 0.4 mm with a gold-plated tip for laser optical reasons to increase safety as well as with additional possibility of aspiration for the vaporized tissue

We initially investigated the fundamental effects of a CO_2 laser (Sharplan) and a neodymium: YAG laser of wavelength 1064 nm on 30 bovine intervertebral discs at different energies both in continuous wave mode and in pulsed mode.

For this purpose, histological workup of the tissue was carried out to delimit the depth of damage. Since suitable light conductor systems which allow certain transmission are not yet available for the CO_2 laser, the further investigations were only carried out with the neodymium: YAG laser. We have developed an introduction instrument for the approach to the intervertebral disc which ultimately has an external diameter of 1 mm and a suitable light conductor with the diameter of 0.4 mm analogous to chemonucleolysis [9–11, 13, 15] (Figs. 1, 2).

In the further course, the investigations were then carried out on bovine tissue with this new instrument set. In a total of 160 bovine intervertebral discs, we then measured the temperature distribution in the disc and in the region of the in situ needle exactly with variation of the impulse duration and energy. In addition, the depth of damage was determined by histological investigations. Finally, the experience obtained and the application of the conditions found to be optimal were initially transferred to six lumbar vertebral movement segments L 4/L 5, L 5/S 1 in human cadaver preparations. Our last step so far was then to extrapolate these results to animal experiments. We placed the needle exactly in a total of 16 intervertebral discs in sheep in the region of the lumbar spine with the percutaneous technique in conjunction with image transducer control, known from chemonucleolysis, and carried out the nucleus pulposus vaporization with the laser in anesthesia. The animals were killed after two weeks, after four weeks and after six weeks, and the tissue was worked up histologically.

Results

We were able to show with our tissue experiments that both the CO_2 laser and the neodymium : YAG laser are entirely able to attain adequate volume effects in the tissue of the nucleus pulposus with open application. However, application with a technique related to that of chemonucleolysis appeared to be necessary to attain a reasonable method which provides advantages both for the patient and the applying physician.

Unfortunately, no reliable light conductors are available at present for the CO_2 laser, so that we were only able to continue our further experiments with the neodymium : YAG laser. After improvement and further development of the introduction instrument and the light conductor for our purposes (see Fig. 2), we then started a systematic investigation of the effects under thermographic control for determination of the temperature distribution. The laser power was varied between 10 and 100 watts in 10-watt steps. The duration of treatment and the duration of pauses was also varied after each shot with single shots from 0.1 second to continuous wave mode. In various series, we were able to allow between 40 and 4000 joules to act on a single preparation.

The contact-free method of measurement of infrared telethermography allowed us to study exactly the temperature distribution, both in space and in time, in the tissue of interest (Fig. 3).

In use of the continuous wave mode, high temperatures were very quickly produced within a few seconds in the intervertebral disc investigated when more than 20 watts were applied. A further disadvantage of the continuous wave mode was that practically only a thin canal was then produced by the laser. In further experiments, we then investigated pulsed methods. With high watt numbers, we only applied very short impulses between 0.1 and 0.5 seconds duration. There are very short-term high temperature peaks at the uncooled tip of the light conductor which vaporize the tissue of the nucleus pulposus directly in fractions of seconds. In thermographic serial investigations, we were then able to establish the conditions shown in Table 1 as definitive. With observation of these conditions, the temperature remains definitively below 40° C even at the annulus fibrosus.

The thermographic method of measurement works continuously, is contact-free, and has high precision. There are 64 000 measurement points in the measurement range. A color thermogram is then generated on the monitor. On the other

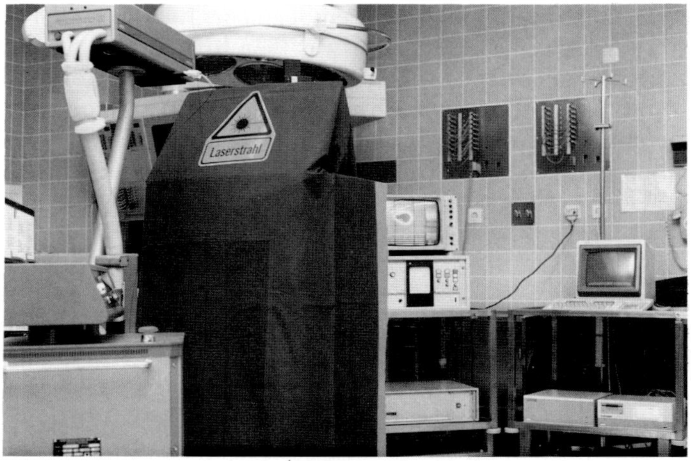

Fig. 3. Experimental design for thermographic measurement with laser, measurement box and thermography camera as well as the pertinent computers which directly process the digital data

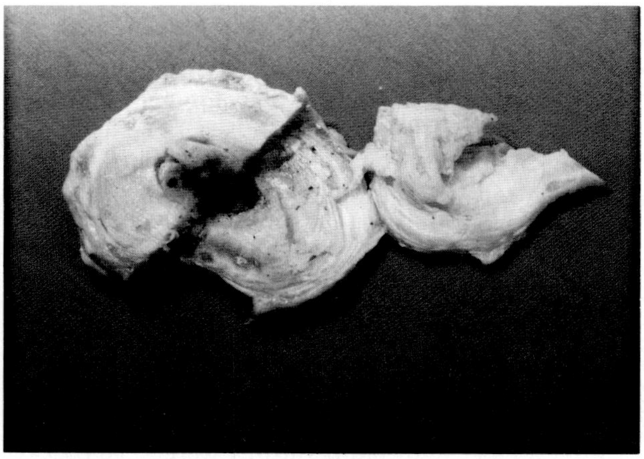

Fig. 4. Intervertebral disc preparation with central vaporization of the nucleus pulposus by laser action (macroscopic)

hand, the digital measurement data are stored in the computer, where they serve as a basis for the further calculations.

After we had established the safe conditions, we investigated the volume dimensions which are to be attained. The scale of the volume effect at the nucleus pulposus depends primarily on the intensity of irradiation (watts per cm^2) in the neodymium: YAG laser (Fig. 4). Via the parameters which can be adjusted on the laser with the head output and total energy which can be determined there, the size of the volume effect can be exactly controlled in an reproducible way. With the given technical possibilities, the adjustment shown in Table 1 has proved effective at present on the basis of the histological evaluations. Figures 5 and 6 show the typical histological appearances of nucleus pulposus vaporization.

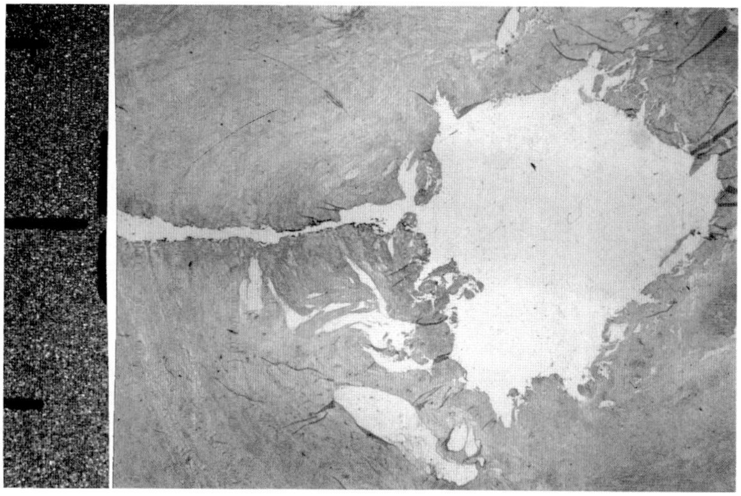

Fig. 5. From the left, hematoxylin-eosin staining of a human intervertebral disc preparation. From the left, the penetration canal, the needle pushed forward with the laser assistance as well as the exactly delimitable volume effect in the nucleus pulposus with minor damage to the marginal zone can be seen

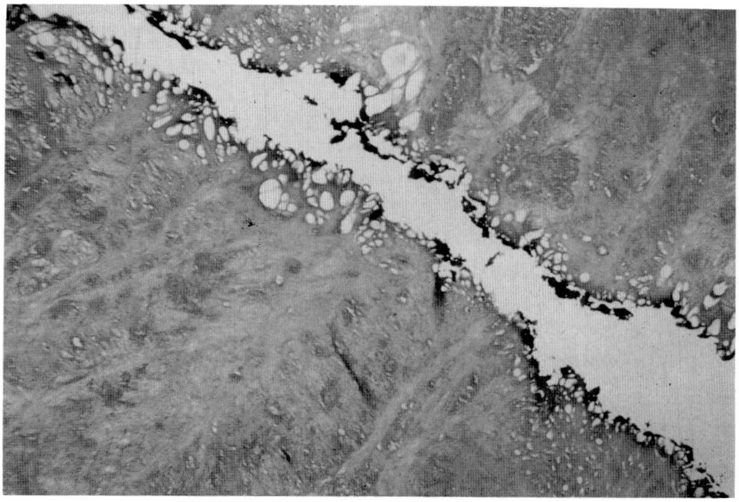

Fig. 6. Enlargement of a detail of the marginal zones with only slight damage and carbonization of the adjacent tissues

Table 1. Neodymium:YAG laser

Wavelength	1064 nm
Single impulse	0.3 seconds
Pause	5 seconds
Output	30 watts
Total	400 to 600 joules

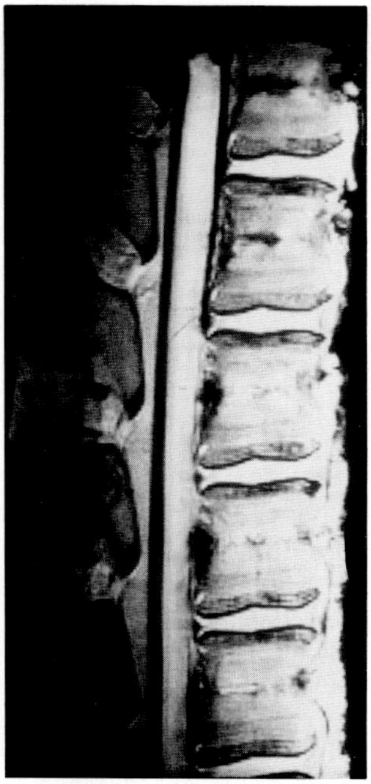

Fig. 7

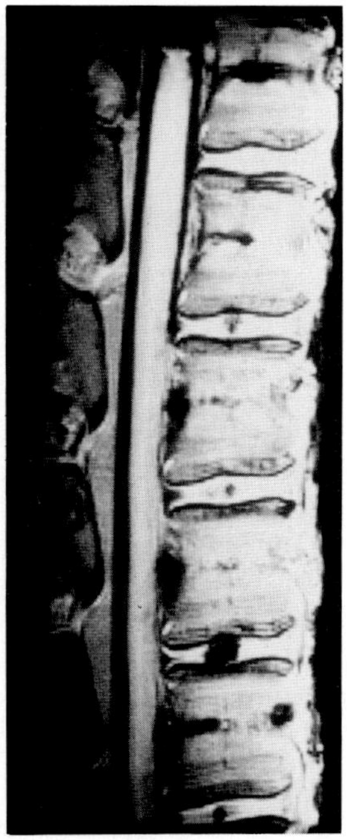

Fig. 8

Fig. 7. Nuclear magnetic resonance tomogram of a lumbar spine before laser application

Fig. 8. Nuclear magnetic resonance tomogram of the same lumbar spine as in Figure 7 from caudal to cranial: chemonucleolysis, laser with conditions as shown in Table 1, chemonucleolysis, laser with conditions for a less pronounced effect

We carried out nuclear magnetic resonance tomographic investigations with special sequences on 10 human spine preparations. The volume effect here can be measured exactly. In these measurements, good constant reproducibility of the effect was also shown. Figures 7 and 8 show a lumbar spine in the NMR tomographic picture before and after laser application. In Figure 8, the effect of a chemonucleolysis can be seen in addition to the laser effects.

A chemonucleolysis and a subsequent laser application under the conditions specified above were carried out here in the lowest intervertebral disc space from caudal to cranial. A chemonucleolysis and, in the uppermost segment, a laser vaporization at lesser intensity were carried out.

In the pictures shown here, freshly prepared discase which had been introduced under image converter control could act for 48 hours before the investigation was carried out. The study of Dolan, Adams and Hutton is referred to with regard to this procedure [6].

Discussion

The technique of nucleus pulposus vaporization with the laser is doubtless still experimental. Owing to its elegant possibilities, however, it deserves an exact examination. This procedure offers a series of important advantages compared to chemonucleolysis, especially in patients with severe pain syndromes. The indication and contraindications as well as intraoperative re-examination of the indication by discography have a basis similar to those in chemonucleolysis, at least at the present time.

In the first instance, a possible indication would be the nonsequestrated lumbar disc prolapse. The fact that an immediate effect which can be controlled with certainty can be attained with the method at the nucleus pulposus with appreciable miniaturization of the instruments can be regarded as advantages of the method.

Anaphylactic reactions as seen in chemonucleolysis are not to be feared, and the problems of nucleotomies following unsuccessful chemonucleolysis, are also avoided. Similar to chemonucleolysis, the method can of course also be carried out under local anesthesia, and this is a particular advantage.

After exact placing of the needle under the image converter, the patient can be asked directly as to the result of nucleus pulposus vaporization. The result must occur immediately. This first experimental experience, which we could also implement definitively in animal experiments, now gives rise to a multiplicity of questions:

What is the appearance of the optical properties of damaged intervertebral discs or of disc prolapse compared to the healthy tissue we have investigated?

How is the biomechanical stability of the spine altered by nucleus pulposus vaporization?

Are there advantages with regard to stability, compared to chemonucleolysis or conventional nucleotomy, since the nucleus pulposus can be removed very selectively?

What are the possibilities offered by other lasers or other wavelengths [1, 7, 12, 16].

We have recently also been able to carry out investigations with a neodymium-YAG laser of the wavelength 1320 nm. A large number of new instruments and also possible light conductors will shortly be suitable for routine use. Perhaps another laser will be even more suitable for this method (alexandrite-holmium-erbium: YAG laser; excimer laser, CO_2 with flexible light conductor).

Finally, a series of investigations in animal models (dachshund with intervertebral disc prolapse) will be necessary to answer the question as to the effectiveness of this therapy in actual intervertebral disc prolapses, not least because of the question of the frequency of recurrences.

Techniques analogous to percutaneous nucleotomy under arthroscopic or bronchoscopic control are being tested (see H. M. Mayer et al., this volume). At all events, the possibility of an elegant, almost conservative form of treatment is available for patients with a nonsequestrated intervertebral disc prolapse with violent sciatica and typical spinal computer tomogram, as well as failure of conservative therapy with nucleus pulposus vaporization. The method has already been introduced clinically in the experimental stage by a study group in New York/Graz [4]. The results are still awaited, but at all events surgical complications have not occurred so far.

References

1. Bellina MD, Joseph H et al. (1984) Analysis of electronically pulsed versus quasi-continuous wave carbon dioxide laser in an animal model. Am J Obstet Gynecol
2. Brinckmann P, Horst M (1985) The influence of vertebral body fracture, intradiscal injection and partial discectomy, on the radial bulge and height of human lumbar discs. Spine 10: 138–145
3. Brinckmann P, Horst M (19869 Short-term biomechanical effects of chymopapain injection: an in-vitro investigation of human lumbar motion segments. Clin Biomech 1: 14–19
4. Choy DSJ, Case RB, Ascher P (1987) Percutaneous laser ablation of lumbar discs. A preliminary report of in-vitro and in-vivo experience in animal and four human patients. 33rd Annual Meeting, Orthopedic Research Society, January 19th–22nd 1987, San Francisco, California
5. Dinstl K, Fischer PL (1981) Der Laser. Springer, Berlin Heidelberg New York
6. Dolan P, Adams MA, Hutton WC (1987) The short-term effects of chymopapain on intervertebral discs. Editorial. British Society of Bone and Joint Surgery, 0030-620X/3102
7. Frank F et al. (1986) Comparative investigation of tissue reaction with 1.06 μm and 1.32 μm Nd: YAG laser radiation. MBB Medizintechnik Ltd., P.O.B. 80 11 68, D-8000 München 80
8. Frank F (1981) Der medizinische Einsatz von Lasern. MBB-AG Information 1/81
9. Fraser RD (1984) Chymopapain for the treatment of intervertebral disc herniation: the final report of a double-blind study. Spine 9: 815–818
10. Görge HH, Curio G, Brock M (1984) Chemonukleolyse als Alternative zur offenen chirurgischen Behandlung des lumbalen Bandscheibenvorfalls. Dtsch Med Wochenschr 109: 68–72
11. Javid MJ, Nordby EJ, Ford LT et al. (1983) Safety and efficacy of chymopapain (chymodiactin) in herniation nucleus pulposus with sciatica. JAMA 249: 2489–2527
12. Müller G, Bader H, Greve P (1985) 9.6 μm-CO_2-Laser für medizinische Anwendungen. Laser 1: 86–88
13. Shepperd JAN (1984) Postero-lateral percutaneous surgery to the lumbar spine. A preliminary report. Royal East Sussex Hospital, Hastings, England
14. Stephen N, Joffe N, Daikuzono, Osborn J et al. (1987) Contact probes for the Nd: YAG laser. Department of Surgery, University of Cincinnati Medical Center, Ohio
15. Suezawa Y, Jacob HAC (1986) Percutaneous nucleotomy. Arch Orthop Trauma Surg 105: 287–295
16. Verhandlungsbericht der Deutschen Gesellschaft für Lasermedizin 1986 (1987) EBM Ltd., München, M2V AG, Zürich
17. Wollenek G, Laufer G, Stangl G, Buchelt M, Wolner E (1986) Thermische Effekte der UV-excimer Laserstrahlung im biologischen Gewebe. Chirurgische Universitätsklinik und Technische Universität Wien

Subject Index

J. Rickenbacher, A. M. Landolt, K. Theiler

Applied Anatomy of the Back

In collaboration with H. Scheier, J. Siegfried, F. J. Wagenhäuser

Translated by R. R. Wilson, D. P. Winstanley

1985. XV, 400 pp. 373 figs., mostly in colour. Hardcover ISBN 3-540-15132-X
Distribution rights for Japan: Igaku Shoin, Tokyo

Over 350 beautifully clear figures combined with precise accompanying text relay an unequivocal picture of the anatomy and function of the back. Both normal anatomy as well as variants and deformations are depicted.
The volume pays special attention to the relationship of the back to other body regions, since back disorders often cause symptoms in other regions and accordingly are of great practical importance. The spinal column and those parts of the nervous system connected with it build the central core of the work. The morphologic fundamentals necessary for an examination are reviewed; in addition the various clinical syndromes which result from the anatomical situation and their diagnosis and treatment are discussed.
For the orthopedic surgeon, traumatologist and neurosurgeon, accesses to the spine, the vascular supply and variants in different body regions, possible complications as well as injuries to the spinal column and cord are comprehensively presented. For the neurologist, rheumatologist and all physicians in the field, this remarkable volume offers an indispensable aid for daily practice.

Springer-Verlag Berlin Heidelberg New York London Paris Tokyo Hong Kong